T

Arthritis Treatment

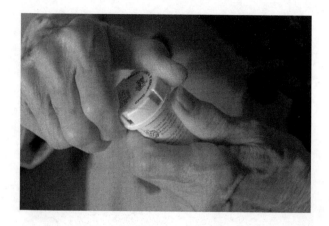

Important stuff you should know to get blessed relief

By

Nathan Wei, MD, FACP, FACR

www.arthritistreatmentcenter.com

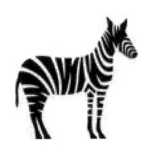

This book should not be a substitute for a thorough examination by your physician. The products that are mentioned in this book are recommended. Prior to using any of them, we recommend you seek advice from a qualified specialist. Neither the publisher nor the author may be held liable for any injury, loss, or damage sustained by anyone who relies on the information contained in the book.

Table of Contents

www.arthritistreatmentcenter.com

www.arthritistreatmentcenter.com

www.arthritistreatmentcenter.com

My doctor has told me I need a joint replacement. What questions do I need to ask?

I have arthritis... What are my options for joint replacement?

Foreword

This book is not meant to be a comprehensive discussion of arthritis.

Rather, the purpose is to highlight some of the more important issues that patients with arthritis often present with in my practice.

This book would not have been possible without the support of my family, staff, and patients.

Let's get started…

Introduction

First off, let's begin with some basic information. The term "arthritis" is derived from Greek…"arthron" meaning " joint" and "itis" meaning inflammation.

Arthritis is a word that refers to more than 100 different conditions!

It is the major cause of physician visits in adults over 65 as well as the most common cause of disability in adults. While that's bad enough, what many people don't realize is that arthritis can cause blindness, paralysis, deafness, and even premature death!

The good news is this: early diagnosis and proper management of arthritis improves both quality as well as quantity of life.

Before I begin, there are some common misconceptions, I'd like to dispel.

> Myth 1:   "Nothing can be done about arthritis..."
>
> The truth is... arthritis when diagnosed and treated properly can be controlled!
>
> Myth 2:   "It's all due to getting old..."
>
> The truth is arthritis affects all age groups including children, teenagers, and young adults. My sister developed rheumatoid arthritis in her thirties and one of my children developed arthritis at the age of ten.

www.arthritistreatmentcenter.com

Myth 3:   "It's just aches and pains... Nothing I can't live with..."

The truth is arthritis is the number one cause of loss of personal freedom. More than 100,000 Americans can't walk independently from their bed to the bathroom because of arthritis!

Myth 4:   I hear this all the time... "What about that stuff I saw advertised on TV. That'll work so why should I see a doctor?

The truth is, most of the things you see advertised on television or in magazines may treat symptoms temporarily but if you happen to have a serious type of arthritis, you're wasting precious time.

Myth 5:   "Arthritis is just a joint disease..."

The truth is, the term arthritis encompasses many conditions such as

- Tendonitis
- Bursitis
- Ligament injuries
- Carpal tunnel syndrome
- Low back and neck pain

And so on.

Plus, many types of arthritis may affect internal organs. These are the situations where a condition that starts out with aches and pains may truly be life-threatening.

www.arthritistreatmentcenter.com

So now that you have a better understanding of what arthritis is… and what it isn't, let's get started…

Chapter 1

Which of these arthritis risk factors do you have?

People often wonder whether that twinge…that new ache or pain might just be a pulled muscle…or could it be arthritis? Naw… it couldn't be… or could it? This article discusses some very well substantiated risk factors you should know about.

While there are more than 100 different types of arthritis, there are some concrete risk factors for some of them that you should be aware of.

Elevated lipids: If you have elevated cholesterol or triglycerides, you may be at risk for developing at least two types of arthritis. The first is osteoarthritis. If your lipids are up the chances are pretty good you're overweight and obesity is a major contributor to the development and worsening of osteoarthritis (OA), the most common type of arthritis. OA typically affects weight-bearing joints such as the neck, low back, hips, and knees. The more weight you're carrying the more pain you'll have. Gout is another type of arthritis that often accompanies elevated lipids. Foods high in cholesterol are usually high in purines, which cause an elevated level of uric acid to accumulate in the blood. Elevated uric acid is a hallmark trait of gout.

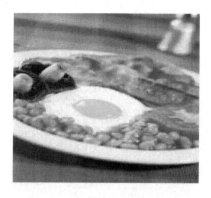

Family history: If you have a family history of any type of arthritis, you are at increased risk for developing that type of arthritis. This is particularly true for diseases such as rheumatoid arthritis, systemic lupus erythematosus, gout, ankylosing spondylitis, and osteoarthritis.

Elevated blood sugar: People with type-2 diabetes often have chronic low grade inflammation. Protein messengers called cytokines are produced. These cytokines – are often associated with inflammatory forms of arthritis.

Obesity: Excessive weight is one of the most common aggravating factors in osteoarthritis.

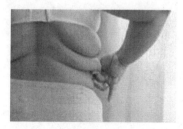

Excessive alcohol intake: Too much beer and red wine can be a trigger for gout. Gout is a type of arthritis caused by excessive production and accumulation of uric acid. In addition, excessive alcohol can harm the liver and lead to harmful effects from abnormal metabolism of drugs such as non-steroidal anti-inflammatory drugs or methotrexate, two types of drugs used commonly to treat arthritis.

Hypertension: Rheumatoid arthritis causes a two-fold increase in coronary heart disease. Associated hypertension aggravates this tendency. In addition, the chances for stroke are dramatically increased in patients with RA. Patients with hypertension also have an increased tendency to develop cardiovascular complications from taking non-steroidal anti-inflammatory drugs.

Smoking: Smoking increases the risk of developing rheumatoid arthritis. It also increases the severity of the disease.

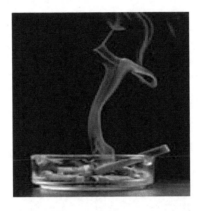

If you have any more than one of these risk factors, do something about them now!

Chapter 2

What are the symptoms of arthritis and what is the treatment?

There are four major arthritis symptoms.

Joint swelling:

Joint swelling, unless it is definitely due to trauma (example: getting tackled in football) may be a symptom of arthritis. The joint will feel tight. Often it will hurt. If the swelling persists for more than a day, it should be evaluated by a physician.

Joint warmth:

When inflammation affects a joint, there will often be warmth in it.

Joint redness:

Along with the warmth, the joint will also have a dusky reddish color. When the joint is warm and red, it will, in most cases, be painful.

Joint pain:

This is the symptom noticed by most people for obvious reasons. While the swelling, redness and warmth may go unnoticed, the pain will not. The pain will vary in intensity. For some people pain will be dull and constant, described as an aching. Others will have sharp shooting pains. The pain may come and go. Sometimes, for example, with osteoarthritis- the pain will cause symptoms at night.

Another is loss of range of motion. This is an inability to move the joint as much as usual.

Stiffness may be a common symptom. This stiffness is most apparent when getting up in the morning or after sitting for a long time during the day.

If any or all of these symptoms persist for longer than a few days, a physician should be consulted. A rheumatologist is an arthritis specialist who will be able to take these symptoms and come up with a specific diagnosis. The diagnosis will determine the treatment needed. Treatment is the subject of another chapter.

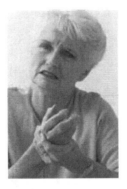

Chapter 3

I have a swollen joint... What kind of arthritis do I have?

When only one joint is inflamed, meaning it has swelling, redness, heat, and pain, the condition is termed "monoarticular arthritis." This means only one joint has arthritis.

There are a limited number of conditions that can cause this problem. They are: trauma, crystal-induced, infection, or tumor.

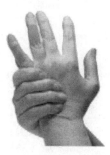

Gout and pseudogout are frequent causes of acute monoarticular arthritis. They are among the most common forms of crystal-induced arthritis. Gout occurs more frequently in men and is rarely seen in premenopausal women. The great toe joint, ankle, and knee are the most commonly affected joints and are usually very painful, swollen, red, and warm.

Conditions such as kidney malfunction and kidney transplantation increase the risk of gout. One major reason, particularly with kidney transplant patients, is the use of drugs such as cyclosporine or tacrolimus.

www.arthritistreatmentcenter.com

Unfortunately, both gout and pseudogout can create a clinical picture where many joints become swollen and inflamed, leading to a misdiagnosis of rheumatoid arthritis.

The diagnosis of gout is confirmed by the presence of monosodium urate crystals in joint fluid. The joint fluid must be examined using a polarizing microscope. That is why it is best looked at in a rheumatologist's office rather than a large commercial lab where the personnel are not used to looking at joint fluid and may not have access to a polarizing microscope.

The joint fluid is inflammatory, with a white blood cell (WBC) count in the 10,000-20,000 range and made up of a specific type of white blood cell called the polymorphonuclear leukocyte. An elevated uric acid is frequently seen, but approximately 30% of patients may have a normal uric acid level at the time of attack.

Pseudogout usually occurs in the elderly and commonly involves the knee, ankle, and wrist. The diagnosis is confirmed by the presence of calcium pyrophosphate dihydrate crystals (CPPD) in an inflammatory joint fluid. The diagnosis is suggested by the presence of chondrocalcinosis on x-ray. Chondrocalcinosis is calcified tissue that often shows up as white lines in the cartilage.

Like gout, the majority of the attacks get better over several days even if untreated. Chronic calcium pyrophosphate dihydrate crystal deposition may occur in the setting of severe osteoarthritis. Sometimes there is a genetic tendency also.

Septic arthritis is always a concern. Septic arthritis refers to a condition where a joint becomes infected with a bacterium.

Patients generally have fever, fatigue, and feel lousy.

The joint is generally warm, red, swollen, and painful.

Gonococcal arthritis, the arthritis due to gonorrhea, is the most common type of septic arthritis. It occurs in sexually active adults. Most patients present with aches and pains that jump from joint to joint, inflamed tendons, and 1 or 2 swollen painful joints. A recent history of sexual exposure is often reported. A peculiar type of skin rash may accompany the aches and pains. The diagnosis is hard to make because the bacteria is hard to culture.

The next most common bacteria are Staphylococcus or Streptococcus. Patients whose immune system is compromised such as alcoholics, diabetics, intravenous-drug abusers, or immunosuppressed patients can be infected with a number of different bacteria.

Any patient with a single inflamed joint should have a joint aspiration using a needle so that the fluid can be analyzed.

Cancers can involve the joint and present as an arthritis affecting one joint. A metastasis (cancer spreading) can result in a severely painful joint.

The diagnosis can frequently be made by imaging either with plain x-rays or magnetic resonance imaging. Biopsy of the lining of the joint arthroscopically (using a small telescope) may be necessary to confirm the diagnosis.

A very peculiar and unusual condition, pigmented villonodular synovitis, is a benign tumor that can result in inflammation of a single joint. This tumor most commonly affects the knee, hip, and finger. Magnetic resonance imaging may be helpful with the diagnosis.

Arthroscopic biopsy may be needed. The treatment is surgical removal of the lining of the joint.

Chapter 4

What is "Inflammatory arthritis?"

There is an old joke. It goes like this: "Neurologists diagnose the untreatable while rheumatologists treat the undiagnosable." Nothing could be truer than when it comes to what is termed "inflammatory arthritis."

Most rheumatologists tend to divide arthritis into two major categories: inflammatory and non-inflammatory. The latter category is also termed "degenerative" arthritis.

The major distinction is that inflammatory types of arthritis have a significant amount of inflammatory cells that attack the joints. These types of arthritis tend to cause more symptoms, particularly stiffness and pain. They also tend to be progressive.

Oftentimes, inflammatory types of arthritis are associated with constitutional symptoms, meaning low grade fever, weight loss, and fatigue. Inflammatory types of arthritis can also cause significant damage to internal organs. Disability and early death may be a consequence of some types of inflammatory arthritis. Examples of inflammatory arthritis are rheumatoid arthritis, systemic lupus erythematosus, psoriatic arthritis, gout, infectious arthritis, and ankylosing spondylitis.

Inflammatory types of arthritis can strike at any age.

Inflammatory types of arthritis have typical patterns although theoretically any joint in the body can be affected.

Inflammatory forms of arthritis may not be easy to categorize. Sometimes it will be obvious that inflammation is present and is a prominent component of the symptom complex. However, a specific diagnosis may not be apparent. Eventually most forms of inflammatory arthritis do "declare" themselves and ultimately fall into a category. But not always! This is a situation where a skilled diagnostician and clinician are worth their weight in gold!

On the other hand, non-inflammatory types of arthritis cause symptoms based on mechanical factors. Often degenerative arthritis affects weight-bearing joints such as the neck, low back, hips, and knees. It tends to occur in older people. While it may progress, it does so relatively slowly. It is rarely, if ever, associated with constitutional symptoms. In fact if constitutional symptoms are present, then either the patient has more than non-inflammatory arthritis or has another illness in addition to their arthritis. This is the type of arthritis people often associate with getting older.

Non-inflammatory types of arthritis may also be confusing sometimes. An example is a condition like fibromyalgia where the pain occurs pretty much all over. Symptomatic and subjective joint swelling may make the clinical diagnosis difficult.

The distinction between inflammatory and non-inflammatory arthritis is made on the basis of a careful history, physical examination, laboratory tests, and imaging procedures such as magnetic resonance imaging (MRI) and ultrasound.

Sometimes a patient can have both types of arthritis. For instance, it is not uncommon for a patient with long standing rheumatoid arthritis to also have degenerative arthritis (osteoarthritis) in a knee or hip.

Interestingly, when an arthroscope (small telescope) is used to visualize the interior of a joint, almost all types of arthritis have an inflammatory component to them. The extent and type of inflammatory change though varies from disease to disease.

The treatment for inflammatory arthritis will vary. While anti-inflammatory medicines are sometimes helpful, it may be necessary to start disease modifying drug therapy. Again the skill and experience of the arthritis specialist is paramount in determining which direction to head. Obviously, if the inflammatory arthritis becomes more well-defined, then treatment becomes easier to define as well.

The key point to remember is that if you do have arthritis, it's important to seek the opinion of an expert arthritis specialist.

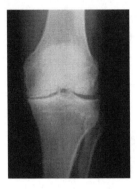

Chapter 5

My rheumatologist says I have "Undifferentiated arthritis" ...what is that?

Among those who seek out a rheumatologist's assistance for joint symptoms are patients who often have a condition called undifferentiated arthritis (UA). This means a specific diagnosis is not yet possible.

Spontaneous remission occurs in 40 to 50 percent of UA patients, while about one-third develop rheumatoid arthritis (RA). Rheumatologists must make a decision regarding whether to initiate disease modifying anti-rheumatic drugs (DMARDS) immediately... or to wait a bit.

To investigate the question as to what could or should be done, researchers with the Early Arthritis Clinic at Leiden University Medical Center, The Netherlands, developed a formula to help determine whether patients who present with UA are likely to progress to RA.

They looked at a total of 1,700 arthritis patients. The Leiden investigators then identified 570 patients with recent-onset UA and monitored their disease for one year. At the end of one year, 177 of the original UA patients fulfilled the diagnostic criteria for RA and 150 had achieved remission; the remaining 94 had been diagnosed with another arthritic condition.

Through a combination of questionnaires, physical examination, and blood samples, the team identified 9 clinical variables with independent predictive value for RA: gender, age, localization of symptoms, morning stiffness, the tender joint count, the swollen joint count, the C-reactive protein level, rheumatoid factor positivity, and the presence of anti-cyclic citrullinated peptide antibodies.

They then created a prediction scoring system.

The prediction score, ranging from 0 to 14, was calculated for every patient in the group, with a higher score indicating a greater risk of developing RA. None of the patients who had a prediction score of less than 3 progressed to RA during the year-long observation. In contrast, all of the patients who had a prediction score of 11 or greater progressed to RA. Among the patients with scores between 4 and 10 who experienced progression to RA, the frequency of such progression increased with rising scores.

The percentage of patients in whom RA developed was also assessed according to several cutoff values of the prediction score. For example, when the scores 5.0 and 9.0 were chosen as cutoff values, 97 percent of patients with UA who had a score equal to or less than 5.0 did not develop RA, and a score of equal to or greater than 9.0 was associated with progression to RA in 84 percent of the patients.

"Because the prediction rule is accurate and can be easily determined in daily clinical practice, the present model is an important step forward in achieving individualized treatment in patients with recent-onset UA," notes chief spokesperson Dr. Tom W. J. Huizinga. "… we believe that the current model allows physicians and patients to make an evidence-based choice regarding whether or not to initiate DMARDs, in the majority of patients presenting with UA."
[van der Helm-van Mil AHM, le Cessie S, van Dongen H, Breedveld FC, Toes REM, Huizinga TWJ. A Prediction Rule for Disease Outcome in Patients With Recent-Onset Undifferentiated Arthritis: How to Guide Individual Treatment Decisions. Arthritis and Rheumatism. 2007: 57 (2).]

Authors note: A version of this prediction scale is already used by practitioners in the United States. By taking into consideration multiple variables, a rheumatologist can usually arrive at a decision about whether to start DMARD therapy or not. One measure that was omitted from the Dutch study that we often use in the U.S. is the use of an imaging procedure such as magnetic resonance imaging (MRI) or ultrasound. These imaging procedures are invaluable for early detection of inflammatory damage (diagnosis) and staging.

We do know that the earlier treatment is started, the more likely a patient will achieve remission. We also know that the more aggressive we are at the beginning of RA, the more likely we are to avoid permanent irreparable damage. On the flip side, the use of strong DMARD therapy or biologic therapy should be tempered with the knowledge that these drugs do have potentially severe side effects.

Chapter 6

Doctor... why does my finger hurt?

Because the hand is involved in so many day-to-day activities, when something goes wrong, the hand problem becomes noticeable quickly.

Fractures and dislocations of the fingers occur as a result of trauma. The diagnosis is pretty easy to make and both the clinical impression as well as x-rays can confirm the diagnosis and prepare the road for treatment.

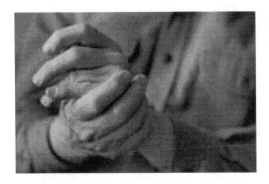

Fingers move as a result of an intricate system consisting of tendons that attach at the near end to muscles in the forearm and hand and at the far end to the tips of the fingers. The tendons run through sheaths that are lined with synovial tissue. The inside of the sheath has a small amount of lubricant that allows smooth movement. In addition, a system of pulleys helps stabilize the tendons. Contraction of the muscles pulls the tendons and allows a person to move their fingers.

A trigger finger is one that locks when the finger is bent. The finger can be straightened only with difficulty. This occurs because the tendon sheath becomes inflamed and narrowed; this inhibits the ability of the tendon to move normally. Injection of an anti-inflammatory medicine (cortisone) usually helps this situation. Ultrasound guided hydrodissection using a small needle to inject a large amount of fluid to release the trigger finger, will often be effective. In rare cases, patients who do not respond to more conservative measures will require surgery.

Another type of painful tendonitis occurs at the outside part of the thumb near the wrist. Activities such as wringing out a rag, and removing lids from jars are very painful. This is called Dequervain's tenosynovitis. Local heat and splinting may help relieve the discomfort. Cortisone injection is often required.

A peculiar form of thickening of the tendon in the palm can lead to a "drawing up" of the third and fourth fingers. This condition- called Depuytren's contracture- occurs most commonly in middle-aged men. It tends to occur in both hands. Surgery is often required. Recently, correction of the deformity using small needles and the use of a new enzyme, have made surgery less likely of an option.

Arthritis can affect the fingers. Specifically, osteoarthritis (OA) can cause painful nodular swelling involving the last row of finger joints-the distal interphalangeal joints. These swellings are called Heberden's nodes. A similar problem in the joints one row in – the proximal interphalangeal joints, is called Bouchard's nodes. These swellings are painful at first. Over time the nodules harden and do not hurt.

Rheumatoid arthritis (RA) is another type of arthritis that affects the hands. The row of finger joints closest to the wrist- the metacarpophalangeal joints is often affected. The proximal interphalangeal joints also are involved in RA.

Gout, pseudogout, and psoriatic arthritis can affect the fingers. Psoriatic arthritis, the arthritis associated with psoriasis, causes a finger to swell up like a sausage. This can be very painful.

Each of these forms of arthritis is treated differently from the other.

Some forms of arthritis such as rheumatoid arthritis and psoriatic arthritis require aggressive therapy.

Finger problems need to be diagnosed properly. In addition to the history and physical exam, x-rays, ultrasound, and magnetic resonance imaging may be required. Once the diagnosis is established, a more precise treatment program can be initiated.

Chapter 7

My wrists hurt... could it be arthritis and what should I do?

Arthritis of the wrist may not sound like a big deal... until you need to open a door, type on your computer, or shake hands. Then you realize how much a role your wrist plays in these simple activities.

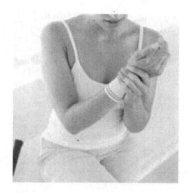

The wrist is like many other joints. It's enclosed in a synovial membrane. It consists of the ends of the radius and ulna- two long bones- that articulate with a row of eight carpal bones. The carpal bones in the wrist also articulate with the metacarpal bones of the hand. The entire wrist complex is stabilized by tendons and ligaments and encased in a synovial membrane.

When arthritis develops, the wrist complex is affected by inflammation of the synovial membrane as well as by any other problem that causes the cartilage that surrounds all the bones in the wrist to wear away.

While wrist pain may occur as the first sign of a problem, the inability to perform simple activities of daily living follows shortly.

www.arthritistreatmentcenter.com

The pain may be dull initially but then becomes sharper and more constant.

Grip strength diminishes. Inflammation progresses, then there may be pressure on the other structures that pass through the wrist such as the median nerve. This leads to carpal tunnel syndrome.

The treatment of wrist arthritis is dependent on the cause. Forms of arthritis that commonly affect the wrist include rheumatoid arthritis, psoriatic arthritis, gout, and pseudogout. When inflammatory forms of arthritis affect the wrist, there is wearing away of cartilage as well as damage to the supporting structures. Wearing away of the cartilage leads to misalignment and deformity as well as wrist dysfunction. Swelling and fluid accumulation may occur.

When wrist arthritis occurs, there is a benefit in that wrist involvement by arthritis generally is often a tip off to diagnosis. For instance, rheumatoid arthritis is one of the more common forms of arthritis that affect the wrist. By allowing an earlier diagnosis, early intervention can lead to remission.

Physical therapy and specific exercise may be beneficial as are splinting and anti-inflammatory medicines. Sometimes, injection with glucocorticoids may be necessary.

In advanced cases, surgery may be necessary. Surgical procedures include excision arthroplasty where the end of the ulna bone is removed. This often helps with some forms of arthritis since it allows more freedom of movement.

Joint fusion and joint replacement may be called for in extreme cases. Wrist replacement currently lasts about ten to fifteen years depending on the amount of activity.

For patients with carpal tunnel syndrome, a new technique using a small needle that is guided by ultrasound to release the median nerve has helped many patients avoid the need for surgery.

Chapter 8

Elbow pain... why does it hurt so much?

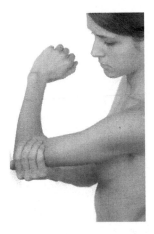

Elbow pain is not often an arthritis problem. Rather, pain is more often due to strain or inflammation involving the supporting structures such as ligaments and tendons.

The elbow is a hinge joint that consists of the articulation of three bones. The olecranon process of the ulna (one of the lower arm bones interacts with the humerus (upper arm bone). The radius (the other lower arm bone) also interacts with the humerus as well as the ulna. As with other joints, the elbow is stabilized by tendons and ligaments and cushioned by bursae.

Inflammatory forms of arthritis such as rheumatoid arthritis, psoriatic arthritis, ankylosing spondylitis, gout, and pseudogout may cause elbow pain and swelling.

Occasionally loose pieces of cartilage can flake off in the joint and cause pain and swelling. The treatment of choice is surgery.

Tendonitis affecting the tendons that allow extension of the wrist is a very common cause of elbow pain. Discomfort is felt at the lateral (outside part of the elbow) and is aggravated by gripping or resisted extension of the wrist. This is known as "tennis elbow."

Tendonitis affecting the tendons that allow flexion of the elbow occurs less often. Pain is felt at the medial epicondyle (inside part of the elbow) and is aggravated by resisted flexion of the wrist. This is also known as "golfer's elbow."

Bursitis can also affect the elbow. Most commonly, bursitis can cause the olecranon bursa (the sac at the tip of the elbow) to become swollen and full of fluid. This can occur as a result of trauma or can also occur as a consequence of inflammatory forms of arthritis such as rheumatoid arthritis or gout.

Entrapment of the ulnar nerve at the elbow (the nerve that causes pain when you hit your "funny bone") can cause pain, numbness, tingling, and weakness involving the 4th and 5th fingers. In severe cases, a "claw hand" may develop.

Trauma can cause fracture.

The history and physical examination almost always point towards the diagnosis.

The laboratory exam is not a valuable part of the work up.

X-rays are helpful for excluding fracture. Magnetic resonance imaging is a more sensitive and specific method of detecting soft tissue abnormalities.

Treatment will vary, depending on whether there is a systemic reason for the elbow problem or not, i.e. if the patient has an inflammatory form of arthritis, that needs to be treated in concert with the elbow problem.

If it is a soft tissue abnormality, effective measures include splints and "tennis elbow bands," anti-inflammatory medicines, and physical therapy. Specific stretching and strengthening exercises are beneficial. For patients who don't respond to these measures, glucocorticoid injection may be helpful.

More recently, a newer form of treatment, percutaneous needle tenotomy is being used. In this procedure, a small needle is used to irritate the damaged tendon. After that is accomplished, platelet-rich plasma (PRP) is injected. PRP contains factors that promote regrowth and healing of the tendon. Ultrasound guidance is needed to ensure accuracy.

When there is fluid inside the joint that causes discomfort or hampers movement, removal of the fluid may be therapeutic. If there is inflammation involving the joint, simultaneous injection of glucocorticoid is indicated.

Since olecranon bursitis sometimes results from infection, fluid drawn from this area should be cultured before steroid injection is considered. Antibiotics are required if infection is the culprit.

Some patients who have refractory pain may need surgery.

Patients with severe arthritis of the elbow may require joint replacement.

Ulnar nerve entrapment can be released using an ultrasound guided needle; this helps patient avoid surgery.

Chapter 9

Doctor... my shoulder really hurts... What do you recommend?

Patients with inflammatory types of arthritis such as rheumatoid arthritis and psoriatic arthritis often have shoulder problems. However, more often than not, a patient presenting with shoulder pain to the rheumatologist will have another reason besides the arthritis for the discomfort they are feeling.

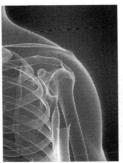

The shoulder is a complicated and complex joint consisting of the interaction of two major bones forming the glenohumeral joint- the joint that joins the upper arm bone to the shoulder blade. The acromioclavicular joint which joins the clavicle (collarbone) to the shoulder blade is also part of this complex. The muscles that help move the shoulder consist primarily of the rotator cuff muscles and their associated tendons: supraspinatus, infraspinatus, subscapularis, and teres minor.

The biceps muscle and tendon are also responsible for shoulder movement as is the deltoid muscle. The shoulder complex is held together via a complicated network of ligaments and tendons that allow the shoulder to have the widest range of motion of any joint in the body. The shoulder complex is surrounded by small fluid filled sacs, called bursae that help to cushion the shoulder joint and allow more purposeful gliding motions of the joint.

Shoulder pain is responsible for about 16% of all complaints having to do with muscles or joints. Shoulder pain becomes defined as being chronic if it lasts 6 months or longer. Age is a general predictor of cause. In patients younger than 40 years, shoulder instability and mild rotator cuff disease are more common. Older patients usually have conditions such as adhesive capsulitis (frozen shoulder), osteoarthritis, and more advanced rotator cuff problems.

Pain located at the top and front of the shoulder is usually due to problems related to the AC (acromioclavicular) joint - that is, the joint that joins the collarbone to the shoulder blade.

By contrast, pain involving the outside of the upper arm near the shoulder joint is often due to bursitis involving the bursa located beneath the deltoid muscle or to tendonitis affecting the rotator cuff.

A diagnosis starts with the history. During the history, the physician will inquire as to the location and duration of pain, whether the pain is present at night, and what types of body positions and movements aggravate the pain.

In addition the range of motion of the shoulder will be assessed. There are two methods for measuring range of motion. Active range of motion is the range of motion a patient can perform on their own. Passive range of motion is what the patient can do with the assistance of the physician.

Problems like tendonitis and bursitis will show that a patient has limited active range of motion but relatively normal passive range of motion.

Loss of both active and passive range of motion suggests adhesive capsulitis or glenohumeral arthritis (arthritis affecting the joint that joins the humerus [upper arm bone] to the scapula [shoulder blade]).

Certain maneuvers designed to "pinch" the rotator cuff against the acromion (the outside part of the shoulder blade) can reproduce the pain in some patients. This condition is called impingement.

Imaging procedures such as x-ray may be helpful in some instances. For example, it can show calcium deposits in tendons or show severe arthritis in the AC joint.

The preferred imaging procedure for suspected rotator cuff disorders is MRI; however, ultrasound is becoming more popular as a cost-effective alternative to MRI. Some studies have indicated that diagnostic ultrasound is actually more precise than MRI for detecting rotator cuff tears.

Conservative treatment is usually initiated for most patients with chronic shoulder pain. This treatment should consist of modification of daily activities such as reduction of overhead activity in patients with rotator cuff disease, glenohumeral osteoarthritis, or adhesive capsulitis.

Cross-body shoulder movements such as swinging a baseball bat, tennis racket or golf club should be limited among patients with AC arthritis.

Non-steroidal anti-inflammatory drugs are frequently used and can be effective.

Injections of glucocorticoids ("cortisone") into the space beneath the acromion are also useful for reducing inflammation. Injections of glucocorticoids directly into the glenohumeral joint are effective in reducing pain and increasing function among patients with adhesive capsulitis. These injections need to be guided using either ultrasound or fluoroscopy to be effective.

Adhesive capsulitis should be treated with a combination of steroid injections as well as physical therapy. Referral to an orthopedist for either manipulation of the shoulder under general anesthesia or arthroscopy is recommended for patients with adhesive capsulitis who do not respond to 2-3 months of therapy.

Osteoarthritis of the glenohumeral joint may respond to NSAIDS and injections into the glenohumeral joint. Physical therapy may also be useful but it should be done gently since too vigorous therapy can aggravate this condition.

Patients with acute massive rotator cuff tears are fairly easy to diagnose and should be referred to an orthopedist as quickly as possible to ensure a good surgical outcome. Massive tears that have been present for 6 weeks or longer are often difficult to repair.

Patients with small tears of the rotator cuff often respond to conservative treatment.

Newer techniques involving the use of percutaneous needle tenotomy (employing a small needle inserted with local anesthetic to "irritate" the tendon to stimulate inflammation) followed by ultrasound guided injection of platelet rich plasma (PRP) to help with the healing process, may allow patients with rotator cuff tears to avoid surgery. This same procedure is being evaluated for arthritis processes as well.

Patients with rotator cuff tears may also respond to stem cell treatment. Stem cells can actually heal rotator cuff tears. This may prevent the need for surgery. Those not responding to more conservative measures can be referred to an orthopedist.

Chapter 10

How to get rid of neck pain simply and easily!

Almost 70 percent of Americans experience neck pain at some point in their lives. Stretching and strengthening exercises have long been considered a key component for keeping the neck strong and healthy.

A Danish study published in 2007 demonstrated that women with neck pain who practiced specific strength training (SST) exercises for the neck and shoulder muscles experienced substantial pain relief.

Neck pain is usually triggered by repetitive use or holding the neck and shoulders, in a poor position as a result of either stress or poor posture habits or both.

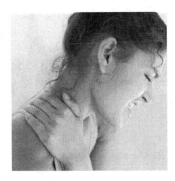

There are many options to consider that can be done simply on your own:

- Stretching exercises. An example is shoulder shrugs. With your arms at the side, breathe in slowly as you shrug shoulders up toward the ears, breathe out as you lower them to a relaxed position. This gentle, repetitive motion works the trapezius muscle in the back of the neck, relaxing this common site of tension. Head tilts also relieve muscle spasms in the neck and increase range of motion. Wrap your right arm around the left side of your head so your right hand is under your left ear. Gently stretch your head toward your right shoulder and count to 10. Repeat on the other side. Try to perform these exercises four to six times each during the day.

- The Danish study focused on dumbbells. These consist of five exercises -- the arm row, shoulder abduction, shoulder elevation, reverse flies and upright row -- targeted toward strengthening the neck and shoulder muscles. Note, however, that in the study these exercises were performed under the close supervision of trainers. If you're interested in giving specific strength training exercises a try, you should contact a personal trainer to teach you how to correctly perform them.

- Take breaks hourly. Long hours at the desk or computer can leave you achy and stiff. Take time once an hour to practice shrugs and head tilts, stretch the muscles and break up the tension. Also, change position frequently. These measures will pay off over the long run.

- Stand (and sit) up straight at all times. Proper posture and alignment of the entire body is critical for ease and comfort in both the neck and back. While sitting, align the base of your spine to the top of your head, with shoulders slightly back and the lower back slightly curved out. While standing, adjust this slightly, now picturing a straight line through your body, into the ground beneath your feet. Place your feet shoulder width apart, bend your knees slightly and find the place where you're neither leaning forward nor backward, but perfectly balanced, with head directly over your feet. If you are doing it correctly, you'll notice less tension in the neck and shoulders.

- Fix your workspace. Little changes can be significant in reducing neck strain and pain. For example, make sure your computer monitor is at eye level... sit up straight with your feet resting comfortably flat on floor... use a chair with armrests that create an angle slightly greater than 90° for your arms.

- Get a headset for your phone. Crooking the phone between your ear and shoulder in order to talk hands-free is one of the worst things you can do to your neck.
- Try self-massage. You can give yourself a pretty good self-massage by putting two tennis balls in a long tube sock. Lie on your back on the floor, rolling these under your shoulder blades and upper back to massage the shoulder blades and break up muscle spasms in the upper back, which connects to the neck muscles.
- Relieve neck pain with heat and cold. When your neck is sore, try a hot pack to soothe the pain... or try a cold pack... whichever feels better.

The treatment of neck pain depends on correctly identifying and addressing its cause, since there are different solutions for muscle pain versus pain from pinched nerves, disk injuries, worn disks or prior trauma.

For neck pain unrelated to stress (such as osteoarthritis), other options such as chiropractic manipulation, ultra high frequency electrical stimulation, gentle horizontal traction using a pneumatic device (similar to a blood pressure cuff), yoga, acupuncture, and massage therapy may be of assistance.

If neck pain persists, more aggressive management may be necessary.

These can include anti-inflammatory drugs, injections of cortisone or lidocaine, botulinum toxin, and rarely surgery.

Chapter 11

Nine little known facts and insider secrets to beating low back pain!

If you have low back pain, then you know how frustrating and agonizing it can be. On top of that, where do you go for treatment? It's so confusing… do you see a physical therapist… A medical doctor… which medical doctor… what about medicines… will I need surgery?

This chapter will give you critical information you must know… so read carefully.

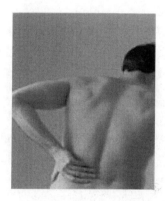

While a ruptured disc is a serious cause of low back pain, it's not the most common cause. Low back pain is usually due to a combination of overuse, muscle strain, and injury to the muscles, ligaments, and discs that support the spine. Over time this leads to an imbalance in the spine.

To make things worse, the causes of pain in the low back tend to add to each other. For example, after straining muscles, you are likely to move in different ways to avoid pain or to use muscles that aren't sore.

This can cause you to strain other muscles that don't usually move that way.

So what can you do? The following are a few suggestions.
Here's where you start...

1. A precise diagnosis is important. A good clinical history and physical exam by an expert is a good start. And imaging procedures such as magnetic resonance imaging (MRI) or computerized tomography (CT) scanning are crucial. Sometimes back pain can be due to unsuspected problems like cancer.
2. Too much rest is bad. Studies have shown that a 24 hour period of bed rest is good for acute low back problems. Longer periods of rest may actually make the situation worse.
3. If you are overweight, you must lose it. There is a multiplication factor involved. You see... an extra pound is more than just an extra pound. For every added pound you carry around your middle there are an extra 5 pounds your back must support!
4. If you are a smoker, STOP. Data has convincingly shown that smokers heal more slowly and prolong the length of time their low back problem persists.
5. Specific exercises designed to stretch and strengthen the low back are an important part of rehabilitation of back disorders. These exercises should be supervised by a skilled physical therapist.

If your back continues to bother you, then...

6. Proper use of anti-inflammatory medicines and muscle relaxants can also be helpful for many patients. Make sure the back doctor you see is experienced in their use because deadly side effects can occur. Injections are helpful but they are also painful and can cause complications!

7. Avoid surgery at all costs! In 1995, researchers conducted an analysis of back surgery procedures, using the 1974 "unnecessary surgery percentage" of 17.6. Testifying before the Department of Veterans Affairs, they estimated that of the 250,000 back surgeries performed annually in the U.S. at a hospital cost of $11,000 per patient, the total number of unnecessary back surgeries approaches 44,000, costing as much as $484 million. (Leape LL. Unnecessary surgery. Health Serv Res. 1989 Aug; 24(3):351-407). There are roughly 900,000 low back surgeries performed annually now. You do the math.

8. Strongly consider internal disc decompression (IDD) for most forms of mechanical low back pain. This is a non-invasive, non-surgical form of back treatment that has up to an 86% response rate. IDD is gentle, effective, and is probably the treatment of choice for most low back disorders.

Finally, some forms of low back pain may be very serious...

9. If you have low back problems and develop numbness and weakness in the legs or loss of bladder or bowel function, you must go straight to the emergency room!!

Chapter 12

Osteoarthritis of the knee... A young person's disease

Osteoarthritis (OA), the premature wearing away of cartilage- the gristle that caps the ends of long bones is the most common form of arthritis. It is the type of arthritis that conjures up the elderly person who has aches and pains.

New data though shows that osteoarthritis probably begins earlier, probably in the second decade, in many patients.

Dr. Ewa Roos, professor in the Institute of Sports Science and Clinical Biomechanics of the University of Southern Denmark, presented an intriguing paper outlining her research. In it she described two populations of patients who suffer from osteoarthritis of the knee. The first group was comprised mainly of older women. The other group, though, consisted of men in their 30's and 40's (Roos EM, et al. Arthritis Rheum 2005; 52: 3507-3514).

A major hurdle to early diagnosis is that many younger patients with symptoms will have negative imaging studies... in other words, x-rays and magnetic resonance imaging (MRI) tests will be normal.

To complicate matters, patients who have x-ray evidence of osteoarthritis don't necessarily have symptoms.

Risk factors that are common to people with osteoarthritis are genetic predisposition and excessive weight.

In addition, patients who have suffered knee injuries to the anterior cruciate ligament (ACL) and menisci- the cartilage cushions in the knee- are also at increased risk for developing OA (Englund M, et al. Arthritis Rheum 2007; 56:4048-4054).

In related studies, it has been shown that regular exercise is both protective and preventative as far as osteoarthritis of the knee is concerned.

In other words, exercise appears to strengthen joint cartilage in patients with OA of the knee. Measurements of glycosaminoglycans, a measure of strength and elasticity in the joint, showed significant improvements in the knees of patients with OA who regularly exercised compared to control subjects who did not.

Many patients with OA of the knees are resistant to the idea of exercise since they feel it may cause the joints to wear down even faster. The results of the above studies clearly indicate that exercise should be encouraged.

For symptomatic relief, strengthening and stretching exercises accompanied by the judicious use of ice and anti-inflammatory medications may be quite helpful.

In the past, corticosteroid ("cortisone") injections were routinely prescribed for patients with moderate to severe pain from OA. However, evidence indicating that corticosteroids ultimately cause cartilage to wear away faster than it should, has concerned physicians to the point where these injections are used less.

Viscosupplements, lubricants that help the knee to glide better, and which may help slow down the process of wear and tear are helpful for some patients.

More recently, the use of autologous stem cell therapy (stem cells harvested from the patient himself) has shown great promise, not only for symptomatic relief but for actual reversal of cartilage wear and tear with possible re-growth of cartilage.

www.arthritistreatmentcenter.com

Total joint replacement is reserved for those patients in whom conservative measures have failed.

Chapter 13

I have arthritis in my ankle... What can I do?

Ankle arthritis is one of the most common problems seen in a rheumatology office. While it is a relatively small joint complex, it is subjected to a great deal of stress because of the weight-bearing required with standing and walking.

Throw in the need to make forward and backward movements as well as side to side movements, it becomes clear that the stress placed on the bones, ligaments and tendons is tremendous. And that doesn't even account for the twisting and pivoting motions that are often required during a typical day.

Because of this responsibility and location, ankles are probably injured more than any other joint complex.

Many different kinds of arthritis can affect the ankle. The most common are osteoarthritis. Osteoarthritis is a wear and tear type of arthritis. The cartilage that cushions the joint begins to wear away prematurely as a result of trauma and localized inflammation. This type of osteoarthritis that occurs following injury is referred to as post-traumatic osteoarthritis. A common scenario is someone who sprains their ankle as an adolescent or young adult and then develops ankle arthritis years later.

Rheumatoid arthritis comprises about 15 percent of ankle arthritis. Rheumatoid arthritis is a chronic systemic autoimmune disease that affects virtually all joints. The chronic inflammation leads to progressive deterioration of cartilage, bone, and ligaments.

www.arthritistreatmentcenter.com

Other types of arthritis that can attack the ankle include psoriatic arthritis, Reiter's disease, gout, pseudogout, sarcoidosis, juvenile arthritis, and ankylosing spondylitis.

Treatment of ankle arthritis first consists of making the correct diagnosis. That takes a careful history and physical examination. Laboratory testing and imaging studies such as x-ray, ultrasound, and magnetic resonance imaging are useful.

Treatment for mild discomfort is straightforward. Limit activities that cause pain. That means high impact sports like running, soccer, and basketball. If excess weight is an issue, then weight loss is mandatory. Over-the-counter anti-inflammatory medicines can also provide symptomatic relief.

Various ankle braces can be a lifesaver. These come in different varieties and shapes. They can fasten using laces or velcro. Braces may be soft or may contain a hard synthetic shell. It is best to consult with your rheumatologist or orthopedist before purchasing a brace.

Orthotics are shoe inserts that tilt the ankle and relieve pain by altering the direction of stress forces. These should be custom-made for optimal results.

Rocker bottom shoes reduce pain with walking because they limit the amount of motion the joint has to go through. People who have had ankle fusion surgery (where the joint is fused together) often find rocker bottom shoes helpful.

When ankle pain is severe due to inflammation and/or fluid accumulation, then aspirating the joint with a needle and injecting a long-acting glucocorticoid ("steroid") may be very useful. Following a procedure like this, it is a good idea for the patient to have their ankle braced for at least three days to rest the joint.

Physical therapy is also an excellent adjunctive therapeutic approach. The therapist can help the patient with different modalities that can reduce edema (soft tissue swelling) as well as inflammation and also teach a patient exercises to strengthen and stabilize the ankle so that future ankle sprains and strains are less likely.

Patients who have severe ankle arthritis due to osteoarthritis may benefit from viscosupplementation. This is a procedure where a lubricant is injected into the joint. Viscosupplements have been used successfully in many joints including the knee, hip, and shoulder, as well as the ankle.

Surgery is an option for patients who have failed more conservative measures. Arthroscopy, which is a procedure where a small telescope is inserted into the ankle joint through a tiny incision, may be suggested. Small instruments are used to remove loose pieces of cartilage. This procedure can also be incorporated with simultaneous cartilage transplant where healthy cartilage is inserted in place of damaged cartilage at the time of the procedure. Cartilage transplant procedures are very time intensive and require limited weight bearing for several weeks to months afterward.

Joint realignment is a procedure where a wedge of bone is removed from one side of the ankle so that stress forces are transferred to the healthy part of the ankle. While this is a temporary fix, it is useful for some patients.

Ankle fusion is a surgical procedure where the tibia (leg bone) is screwed to the talus (upper ankle bone). This restores alignment and reduces pain. Unfortunately, the patient loses about half of the plantar and dorsiflexion (toe down and toe up) movement in the ankle. The ability to walk without pain is restored to the ankle; however, there is more stress placed on other weight-bearing joints such as the knee, which can lead to the development of osteoarthritis in these joints.

Ankle replacement is an increasingly popular option. In the past, ankle replacements weren't that effective but technological advances have improved their success. Good candidates for ankle replacement are those who are older than 55 years of age, in good medical condition, have their weight in the normal range, and who don't engage in high impact activities either at work or during their leisure time.

Chapter 14

Foot pain relief at last!

As an arthritis specialist, one area that I see people complain about more often than almost any other, is their feet. This is too bad because there are many treatments that can be helpful.

The foot is made up of 26 bones and 39 muscles...

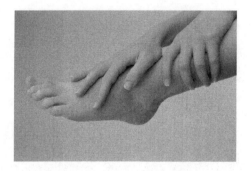

The foot and ankle are designed to bear weight. The multiple joints in the feet are capable of adjusting to almost any terrain and the padding in the feet are designed to absorb shock. The ankle joint allows the foot to move up and down, side to side, and inward and outward (inversion and eversion).

Not All Foot Pain Comes From The Foot!

Careful examination of the low back, hip, and knee should be performed because pain from these areas may affect the foot and ankle. In particular, pinched nerves in the low back can cause foot pain and weakness.

www.arthritistreatmentcenter.com

Ankle sprains are common- 25,000 people sprain an ankle every day! The goal of treatment is to relieve pain and prevent instability. Treatment of an acute sprain consists of rest, ice compression and elevation ("RICE"). Exercises to help stabilize and strengthen the ankle should be started.

Arthritis of the ankle may cause recurrent pain and swelling. Pain from arthritis typically is made worse by weight-bearing particularly on uneven ground. What this means is you should try to avoid excessive walking or running on uneven ground. Anti-inflammatory medication and proper foot support can do wonders.

Pain in the ball of the foot has many causes...

- Foot strain occurs when a person "overdoes it." And the treatment is pretty straightforward. Rest.
- Morton's neuroma (a benign nerve tumor usually located between the 3rd and 4th toes).
- Tarsal tunnel syndrome (pinched nerve in the ankle).
- Arthritis.

Other common causes of foot pain include:

- Stress fractures may occur after excessive walking.
- Achilles tendonitis causes pain in the back of the heel. Treatment consists of anti-inflammatory medicines, rest, a heel lift, and gentle stretching.
- Plantar fasciitis causes pain in the bottom of the heel. Treatment includes rest, anti-inflammatory medication, heel cup, orthotics, stretching, and local steroid injection.
- Flat foot.

Muscle strengthening exercises and orthotics are helpful. Two other common problems are:

- Osteoarthritis, particularly common in the big toe. The big toe will point out to the side. When bursitis alongside the great toe joint develops, this condition is referred to as a bunion. Treatment involves proper padding and footwear. In extreme cases, surgery is required.
- Neuropathy. This painful condition is particularly common in diabetics. This occurs when the small nerves in the feet are damaged. Symptoms include burning, tingling, and pain in the feet - worse at night.

Well fitted orthotics (arch supports) can alleviate not only foot and ankle pain but pain in the knees, hips, low back, and neck!!

We often take the ability to walk for granted. This ability involves the use of two engineering marvels- our feet and ankles. Because of the tremendous amount of force transmitted to the feet with walking, unique problems may develop. Attention to proper preventative care, i.e., comfortable shoes, socks, hygiene, support, along with proper prompt medical care can really put the brakes on foot pain.

Chapter 15

How experts erase heel pain!

The diagnosis of heel pain is best done by looking at the location of the pain... "Where does it hurt?"

Heel pain can occur in two major locations: the back of the heel and the bottom of the heel.

Pain at the back of the heel has three major causes.

Achilles tendonitis is the most common. It is usually the result of injury or overuse. An example is the weekend warrior who decides to go out and run 4 or 5 miles going up hills... or a person who goes on a long walk in flat shoes, shoes with little or no heel. In both cases, stress is placed on the Achilles tendon- the large thick cord located in the back of the heel.

This tendon- the largest in the body- connects the gastrocnemius (calf) muscle to the back of the heel.

The likelihood of Achilles tendonitis developing is increased if a person has flat feet. Older patients taking corticosteroid medications and people treated with quinolone antibiotics like ciprofloxacin (Cipro) also are at increased risk of Achilles tendonitis and even Achilles tendon rupture.

Haglund's syndrome presents with a bony bump located at the back of the heel. A bursa (small sack of fluid) located near the bump may contribute to the swelling. The Achilles tendon insertion near the bony swelling may become inflamed. Because of the location, this syndrome is often referred to as "pump bumps" and the cause often attributed to women's shoes.

Inflammation of the Achilles tendon at its insertion into the heel can be seen with certain types of arthritis, specifically the spondyloarthropathy group which consists of Reiter's disease, psoriatic arthritis, and ankylosing spondylitis. Other signs of disease such as low back pain and stiffness, rash, and joint swelling may provide clues to diagnosis.

Pain in the bottom of the heel is usually due to plantar fasciitis.

Pain in the plantar fascia presents with a sharp stabbing pain in the bottom of the heel. Plantar fasciitis is a common problem that is due to repetitive trauma to the soft tissue in the heel.

Typically a patient will feel fine so long as they are lying down or sitting. But if they get up to walk, the pain feels like an ice pick is being jammed into the bottom of the heel.

This pain gets better over several minutes but occurs again after inactivity followed by weight-bearing.

Causes of plantar fasciitis include:

- An abrupt increase in activity
- Worn footwear
- Footwear with no arch support (e.g. flip-flops)
- Obesity
- Recent rapid weight gain such as with pregnancy
- Overuse as in excessive running and over-training
- Systemic inflammatory arthritis (particularly ankylosing spondylitis and other spondyloarthropathies such as Reiter's disease and psoriatic arthritis)

Treatment involves first establishing the diagnosis. Most of the time, the diagnosis can be suspected by the history and physical examination.

www.arthritistreatmentcenter.com

Imaging tests such as diagnostic ultrasound and magnetic resonance imaging can confirm the diagnosis, if necessary. X-rays may reveal the presence of a heel spur. A heel spur, by itself, is not the cause of pain in the bottom of the heel and heel pain should not be attributed to "a heel spur".

Once the diagnosis has been made, treatment options include:

- Identifying likely causative factors such as excessive weight, inappropriate footwear, and errors in training.
- Non-steroidal anti-inflammatory drugs (NSAIDs) sometimes provide symptomatic relief.
- Therapeutic taping gives short-term symptom relief.
- Exercises to stretch the heel cord and plantar fascia.
- Orthotic devices can help in the short-term reduction of pain. These can be off-the-shelf or custom made. For people with Achilles tendonitis, having the patient wear a lift in the shoe to elevate the heel will help reduce symptoms.
- Glucocorticoid (steroid) injection may also work for plantar fasciitis; however, I don't recommend it since steroids will cause atrophy of the heel pad. I do recommend a procedure called percutaneous needle tenotomy (poking small holes in the plantar fascia and then injecting platelet-rich plasma (PRP). Diagnostic ultrasound should be used to guide blockade of the tibial nerve before the procedure for regional anesthesia as well as to guide the needle for the tenotomy and PRP.

Caution should be observed with the Achilles tendon as far as steroid injection. The tendon can be weakened if steroids are directly injected. This then can lead to Achilles rupture.

For chronic Achilles tendonitis, the procedure of choice is definitely percutaneous needle tenotomy followed by ultrasound guided injection of PRP.

The bursitis that occasionally accompanies Achilles tendonitis (retrocalcaneal bursitis) will respond to steroid injection… and in chronic cases, PRP.

If a patient is taking a quinolone antibiotic (such as ciprofloxacin), it should be discontinued and the patient should be monitored for tendonitis and tendon rupture.

Night time braces are sometimes used for plantar fasciitis.

Often the best treatment for heel pain, whether it is located in the back or on the bottom, is rest.

A surgical solution should be considered for those patients with intractable pain which remains despite conservative treatment.

Chapter 16

I hurt all over... what's wrong with me?

Probably the most common cause of widespread aches and pains is a self-limited viral infection. Nonetheless, a specific diagnosis is necessary before effective treatment can be recommended.

In most cases, a list of possible causes can be established by history and physical examination and a few simple tests. The latter are recommended when symptoms are severe or have lasted longer than 1 or 2 weeks. Extensive testing should be reserved for situations when the clinical diagnosis is unclear.

In an arthritis specialist's office, the following conditions are what are generally encountered.

Fibromyalgia (FM) affects about two percent of the population and can start at any age; it is more common in women than in men. By the time the diagnosis is made, patients have often had symptoms for many months to years. Patients with fibromyalgia complain of pain all over and, by definition, have pain on both sides of the body, above and below the waist, and in both the trunk and extremities.

Patients describe the pain in many different ways. Muscle stiffness is a very common complaint. Other features include non-restorative sleep, meaning the patient wakes up feeling as if they haven't slept, irritable bowel syndrome, irritable bladder, headaches, numbness and tingling in the hands and feet, a sensation of swelling of the hands and feet, and hypersensitivity to sensory stimuli such as smells, sounds, and lights. Fibromyalgia is frequently associated with depression, memory and concentration difficulties, and anxiety, and it often accompanies other chronic painful disorders.

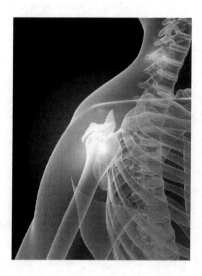

A diagnosis of fibromyalgia is made when there is widespread pain lasting for at least 3 months accompanied by tenderness at discrete locations. The exact location of these tender points forms the basis of the American College of Rheumatology diagnostic criteria for the diagnosis of FM. Patients with fibromyalgia are often tender all over; the presence of tenderness other than at the classic locations does not exclude the diagnosis.

A diagnosis of fibromyalgia does not mean that further tests are not required. The diagnosis of FM is a diagnosis of exclusion, meaning all other conditions that could be present need to be ruled out. A physician should make the diagnosis of FM with reluctance in an older patient without a long history of musculoskeletal symptoms. The cause of fibromyalgia is unknown, and its relation to preceding trauma, such as motor vehicle accidents, is controversial.

Current approaches to treatment include a comprehensive and integrated combination of the use of selective serotonin and nor-epinephrine uptake inhibitors (SSRIs, SSNIs), cognitive behavioral therapy, and non-impact aerobic exercise.

Inflammatory muscle diseases (myopathy) such as dermatomyositis and polymyositis, typically cause muscle weakness rather than pain, although pain is sometimes prominent, especially if there is associated joint inflammation. A careful history and examination will usually permit the physician to distinguish between true muscle weakness and weakness due to pain. Muscle pain may be significant in disorders due to toxins or drugs such as cholesterol-lowering agents or colchicine. Hypothyroidism sometimes presents as a myopathy, with muscle weakness and an elevated creatine phosphokinase (CPK) level, or as generalized muscle pains with normal muscle enzymes.

In the elderly, rheumatoid arthritis may start with typical generalized aches and pains accompanied by an elevation in the erythrocyte sedimentation rate (ESR). Symmetrical joint swelling, particularly involving the small joints of the hands, feet, and wrists may then appear weeks or months later.

Polymyalgia rheumatica (PMR) is a disorder affecting people over the age of 50 years. It is characterized by the presence of inflammation in joints. Patients with PMR have widespread pain and stiffness, which is most severe in the neck, hips, thighs, and low back. Other symptoms such as fatigue, malaise (feeling lousy), fevers and weight loss are often prominent and may actually override the musculoskeletal complaints. Fatigue and malaise can lead to a mistaken diagnosis of depression. Physical findings include pain with movement of the shoulders, hips and knees; some patients cannot raise their arms over their head because of the pain. There may be joint swelling involving the fingers, wrists and knees.

Laboratory tests will often show anemia, an elevated platelet count, an erythrocyte sedimentation rate (ESR) of over 40 mm/h, and elevated liver enzymes in up to one third of patients. Results will be negative for rheumatoid factor and anti-nuclear antibodies. Although most patients will have a markedly elevated ESR, roughly 20 percent of patients can have a pretreatment ESR of 30 mm/h or lower.

Giant cell arteritis (GCA) is a disorder due to inflammation of medium and large blood vessels that typically involves arteries of the head and neck. GCA and PMR are closely related disorders that may develop together or one may precede the other. In addition to the constitutional symptoms associated with PMR, symptoms of GCA include headache, swelling of the temporal artery, scalp tenderness, jaw cramping with chewing, tongue or throat pain and visual disturbances.

Physical findings are variable for this condition. When this diagnosis is suspected, the patient should be sent for a temporal artery biopsy and started on high doses of corticosteroids immediately because of the risk of sudden blindness associated with untreated GCA. A temporal artery biopsy should be done for all other patients with suspected GCA. It is sometimes necessary to do bilateral temporal artery biopsies to prove the diagnosis. A temporal artery biopsy can be performed within one to two weeks of starting treatment without compromising the biopsy findings.

Occasionally, a patient with mild symptoms of PMR may be successfully treated with non-steroidal anti-inflammatory drugs (NSAIDs). However in most cases, low dose prednisone is required. A usual course of therapy for PMR begins with prednisone, 10-20 mgs as a single morning dose. Patients with PMR usually require treatment with corticosteroids for extended periods, often for at least 18 months. Gradual tapering is required. Attempts to reduce prednisone doses more quickly may lead to a flare-up of symptoms; therefore, it is best to taper at a rate that will have patients off the drug in no less than 12-18 months. Alternate-day corticosteroids are usually poorly tolerated and should not be used.

The treatment of GCA usually requires higher initial doses of prednisone, usually 40–60 mg daily in divided doses, to reduce the risk of sudden blindness.

As with PMR, patient symptoms and changes in the ESR are used to guide tapering. The ESR often rises gradually as the prednisone dose is reduced. A sudden rise in the ESR should raise suspicions regarding recurrence of disease, as well as alternative causes, such as infection. A rise in the ESR without associated symptoms is not an indication for increasing the dose of corticosteroid; however, it may delay further dose reductions. Evidence of disease flare-ups should lead to an increase in the prednisone dose to suppress symptoms and reduce the ESR. Corticosteroid treatment is usually continued for at least a year. Steroid-sparing agents such as azathioprine or methotrexate are occasionally helpful in patients who are unable to tolerate reductions in prednisone.

The prolonged use of corticosteroids is typically associated with multiple side effects, including osteoporosis, weight gain, hypertension and glaucoma.

Paget's disease of bone is another condition that can cause aches and pains. The diagnosis can often be suspected because of an elevation of blood alkaline phosphatase and confirmed by x-ray along with bone scan or magnetic resonance imaging. Untreated Paget's disease can lead to severe deformity and in rare cases, congestive heart failure. The treatment involves the use of bisphosphonate drugs.

Various malignancies, both primary as well as metastatic need to be considered in the list of potential causes of generalized aches and pains. Any tumor that can metastasize to bone is suspect. Also leukemia, lymphoma, and multiple myeloma need to be excluded.

In the final analysis, a patient who aches all over is a challenging problem for the clinician. A careful history, physical examination, and further testing can usually lead to the diagnosis.

www.arthritistreatmentcenter.com

Chapter 17

I have arthritis that affects a lot of my joints... Could it be rheumatoid arthritis and how will the doctor know what it is?

There are more than 100 different kinds of arthritis. Most of them involve inflammation. When a patient goes to a rheumatologist to get a diagnosis, there is a process of elimination in order to arrive at the proper diagnosis. This process of elimination is called "differential diagnosis."

Differential diagnosis can be a difficult undertaking because so many forms of arthritis, particularly inflammatory forms of arthritis look alike. The following is a list of types of inflammatory arthritis that can be seen and must be considered when evaluating a patient with inflammatory symptoms of arthritis.

Rheumatoid Arthritis (RA)

RA is a chronic, autoimmune, inflammatory disease that may affect any joint in the body but preferentially attacks the peripheral joints (fingers, wrists, elbows, shoulders, hips, knees, ankles, and feet). It can also affect non-joint organ systems such as the lung, eye, skin, and cardiovascular system. The onset of RA may be insidious-slow-with nonspecific symptoms including fatigue, malaise, loss of appetite, low-grade fever, weight loss, and vague aches and pains, or it may have an abrupt onset with inflammation involving multiple joints. The joint symptoms usually occur bilaterally and are symmetric. Damage to joints- called "erosions" can be seen with magnetic resonance imaging early on or by x-ray later in the course of disease. Approximately 80%

of patients with RA will have elevated levels of rheumatoid factor (RF) or anti-CCP antibodies.

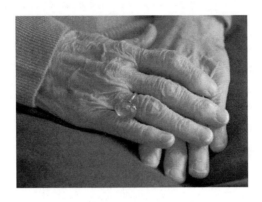

Juvenile Rheumatoid Arthritis (JRA)

JRA describes a group of arthritic conditions that occur in children under the age of 16. Three forms of JRA exist, including oligoarticular (1-4 joints), polyarticular (> 4 joints), and systemic-onset or Still's disease. The latter is associated with significant internal organ involvement and may also present with fever and rash in addition to joint disease. Polyarticular JRA is considered to be the type that is most similar to adult RA, and is responsible for approximately 30% of cases of JRA. Most children with polyarticular JRA are negative for RF and their prognosis is usually good. Roughly, 20% of polyarticular JRA patients will have elevated RF, and these patients appear to be at more risk for chronic, progressive joint destruction and damage. Uveitis- an inflammatory condition of the eye- is a common finding in oligoarticular JRA, especially in patients who are anti-nuclear antibody (ANA) positive. The dangerous feature of uveitis is that it can cause relatively few symptoms so careful screening is recommended in order to avoid blindness.

Systemic Lupus Erythematosus (SLE)

SLE is a chronic inflammatory autoimmune disorder that can involve the skin, joints, kidneys, brain, and blood vessel walls. At least 4 of the following symptoms which have been formulated by the American College of Rheumatology are generally present for a diagnosis to be made:

- Red, butterfly-shaped rash on the face, affecting the cheeks;
- Typical skin rash on other parts of the body;
- Sensitivity to sunlight;
- Mouth sores;
- Joint inflammation (arthritis);
- Fluid around the lungs, heart, or other organs;
- Kidney dysfunction;
- Low white blood cell count, low red blood cell count due to hemolytic anemia, or low platelet count;
- Nerve or brain dysfunction;
- Positive results of a blood test for ANA; and
- Positive results of a blood test for antibodies to double-stranded DNA or other antibodies including anti-Smith antibodies or antiphospholipid antibodies.

Patients with lupus can have significant inflammatory arthritis. That is why lupus can be difficult to distinguish from RA, especially if other signs and symptoms of lupus are minimal.

Inflammatory Muscle Disease

Polymyositis (PM) and dermatomyositis (DM) are types of inflammatory muscle disease. These conditions typically present with bilateral (both sides) large muscle weakness. In the case of DM, rash can be a presenting sign. Diagnosis consists of four major features, including elevation of creatine kinase (CPK), signs and symptoms such as muscle weakness, elevated muscle enzymes (creatine kinase, aldolase), electromyograph (EMG) abnormalities, and a positive muscle biopsy. Often, laboratory test abnormalities can be seen including the presence of autoantibodies such anti-nuclear antibody (ANA), and the myositis-associated antibodies.

In both PM and DM, inflammatory arthritis can be present and can look like RA -- including lung involvement. In RA, however, unless an overlap syndrome – i.e. a patient having both RA as well as muscle disease) is present, muscle function should be normal. Also, in PM and DM, erosive joint disease is unlikely. RF and anti-CCP antibodies are typically elevated in RA and not PM or DM.

Spondyloarthropathies (SA)

A group of arthritic conditions called the spondyloarthropathies which include psoriatic arthritis, reactive arthritis, ankylosing spondylitis, and enteropathic arthritis are a category of diseases that cause inflammation throughout the entire body, particularly in parts of the spine and at other joints where tendons attach to bones. They also can cause pain and stiffness in the neck, upper and lower back, tendonitis, bursitis, heel pain, and fatigue. They are often called seronegative arthritis. The term 'seronegative' means that tests for lab markers such as rheumatoid factor are negative. Symptoms of adult SA include:

- Back and/or joint pain;
- Morning stiffness;
- Tenderness near bones;
- Sores on the skin;
- Inflammation of the joints on both sides of the body;
- Skin or mouth ulcers;
- Rash on the bottom of the feet; and
- Eye inflammation.

In some cases of SA, peripheral arthritis resembling RA can be present. Careful history and physical examination can usually distinguish between these syndromes, especially if an obvious disease that is aggravating inflammation is present (psoriasis, inflammatory bowel disease). In addition, since RA rarely affects the end joints of the fingers (DIP joints), if these joints are involved from inflammatory arthritis, the diagnosis of an SA is favored. Usually, RF and anti-CCP antibodies are negative in SA, although in some cases of psoriatic arthritis there may be elevations of RF and anti-CCP antibodies.

Crystal Associated Arthritis

Monosodium Urate Disease (Gout)

Gout is due to deposition of monosodium urate crystals in a joint. Gouty arthritis is typically sudden in onset, very painful, with signs of significant inflammation on exam (red, warm, swollen joints). Gout can affect almost any joint in the body, but typically affects "cooler" regions including the toes, feet, ankles, knees, and hands. Diagnosis is made by withdrawing fluid from a joint and examining the fluid under a polarizing microscope. Patients may also have elevated serum levels of uric acid.

In most cases, gout is an acute disease that affects one joint and is easily distinguished from RA. However, in rare cases, chronic erosive inflammation can develop and affect multiple joints. And, in cases where tophi (deposits of uric acid under the skin) are present, it can be difficult to distinguish from erosive RA. However, crystal analysis of joints or tophi and blood tests should be helpful in distinguishing gout from RA.

Calcium Pyrophosphate Deposition Disease (CPPD; Pseudogout)

CPPD disease is caused by deposits of calcium pyrophosphate dehydrate crystals in a joint. The body's reaction to these crystals, leads to significant inflammation. Diagnosis includes:

- Detailed medical history and physical exam;

www.arthritistreatmentcenter.com

- Withdrawing fluid from a joint using a needle;
- Joint x-rays to show crystals deposited on the cartilage (chondrocalcinosis);
- Blood tests to rule out other diseases (e.g., RA or osteoarthritis).

In most cases, CPPD arthritis presents with acute arthritis affecting one or more joints. However, in some cases, CPPD disease can present with chronic symmetric multiple joint erosive arthritis similar to RA. RA and CPPD disease can usually be distinguished by joint fluid examination demonstrating calcium pyrophosphate crystals, and by blood tests, including RF and anti-CCP antibodies, which should be negative in CPPD arthritis.

Sarcoid Arthritis

Sarcoidosis is an inflammatory type of arthritis. The majority of patients with this disease have lung disease, with eye and skin disease being the next most frequent signs of disease. In most cases, the diagnosis of sarcoidosis can be made on clinical and x-ray presentation alone. Patients will have acute arthritis, painful nodules under the skin on the shins (erythema nodosum), and a chest x-ray showing enlargement of lymph nodes. In some cases, the demonstration of a specific type of inflammation change, called a non-caseating granuloma on tissue biopsy, is necessary for definitive diagnosis.

Arthritis can be present in approximately 15% of patients with sarcoidosis, and in rare cases can be the only sign of disease. In acute sarcoid arthritis, joint disease is usually rapid in onset, symmetric, involving the ankle joints. The knees, wrists, and small joints of the hands can be involved. In most cases of acute disease, lung and skin disease are also present. Chronic sarcoid arthritis typically involves one or maybe a few joints and due to its often erosive nature can be difficult to distinguish from RA.

Polymyalgia Rheumatica (PMR) / Temporal Arthritis

PMR is a form of arthritis that leads to inflammation of tendons, muscles, ligaments, and tissues around the joints. It is characterized by large muscle (shoulders, hips, thighs, neck) pain, aching, morning stiffness, fatigue, and in some cases, fever. It can be associated with temporal arteritis/giant-cell arteritis (TA/GCA) which is a related but more serious condition in which inflammation of large blood vessels can lead to complications such as blindness, aneurysms and cramping pain in the arms or legs (limb claudication) due to inflammation and narrowing of the large blood vessels in the chest and extremities. PMR is diagnosed when the clinical picture is accompanied by elevated markers of inflammation (ESR and/or CRP). If temporal arteritis is suspected (headache, vision changes, limb claudication), biopsy of a temporal artery may be necessary to make the diagnosis.

PMR and TA/GCA can present with symmetric inflammatory arthritis similar to RA. These diseases can usually be distinguished by blood tests. In addition, headaches, acute vision changes, and large muscle pain are uncommon in RA, and if these are present, PMR and/or TA/GCA should be considered.

Infectious Arthritis

Many infections can present with arthritis either due to direct joint infection or due to autoimmune joint inflammation. In most cases, infections lead to acute single joint arthritis; however, in some cases, chronic arthritis affecting a few or many joints can be present. Because missed infections can lead to significant complications, it is crucial to have a high index of suspicion for infection in any patient presenting with acute or chronic arthritis.

Lyme disease

Lyme disease is an infection due to a type of bacteria called a spirochete. The disease is manifested by a skin rash, swollen joints and flu-like symptoms, caused from the bite of an infected tick. Symptoms may include:

- A skin rash, often resembling a bulls-eye (target lesion);
- Fever;
- Headache;
- Muscle pain;
- Stiff neck; and
- Swelling of knees and other large joints.

The diagnosis of Lyme disease is typically made by blood testing. If, however, chronic single joint arthritis develops, joint fluid analysis or joint tissue biopsy may be necessary for diagnosis. Lyme arthritis can usually be distinguished from RA by clinical presentation and blood tests.

Acute rheumatic fever (ARF)

Acute rheumatic fever is an inflammatory disease that may develop after an infection with the Streptococcus bacteria (strep throat or scarlet fever). The disease can affect the heart, joints, skin, and brain. Symptoms include:

- Fever;
- Joint pain;
- Arthritis (mainly in the knees, elbows, ankles, and wrists);
- Joint swelling;
- redness or warmth;
- Abdominal pain;
- Skin rash
- Skin nodules;
- A peculiar movement disorder (Sydenham's chorea)
- Nosebleeds;
- Heart problems, which can be asymptomatic.

The diagnosis of ARF is made by clinical assessment and blood testing for antibodies against streptococcal proteins. ARF and RA can have similar clinical features including arthritis and nodules. However, ARF can usually be distinguished from RA by clinical presentation. Rash and migratory arthritis are unusual in RA. The use of blood tests is also helpful.

Viral arthritis (hepatitis B and C, parvovirus, EBV, HIV)

Arthritis may be a symptom of many viral illnesses. This makes viral infections a great masquerader. The duration is usually short, and it usually disappears on its own without any lasting effects. Clinical features in adults:

- Joint symptoms occur in up to 60%. These can be symmetric and affect the small joints of the hands, wrists, and ankles as well as the knees. Morning stiffness is also present.
- Parvovirus B19 is a very common viral infection that looks like RA.
- Diagnosis of viral arthritis is made by serologic testing. A high percentage of patients with hepatitis C may have elevated titers of RF. Therefore, RF testing is not helpful in distinguishing between hepatitis C infection and RA. However, in these situations, testing for anti-CCP can be helpful as anti-CCP antibodies have not been shown to be significantly elevated in isolated hepatitis C infections.

So as you can see... "it ain't easy..."

Chapter 18

Doctor... Why is my arthritis worse when the weather changes?

Patients with arthritis often claim that their symptoms are affected by the weather. While most academic rheumatologists discount this phenomenon citing numerous studies, I have a different opinion. And that opinion has been supported by research and experience.

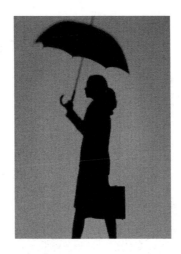

One study from Argentina looked at a group of 183 people; 151 with arthritis (rheumatoid arthritis, osteoarthritis, fibromyalgia) and 32 people without arthritis. Participants were asked to keep a journal for a year recording factors such as barometric pressure, relative humidity, and temperature along with symptoms on a daily basis. Patients with all three types of arthritis experienced more pain on days when the temperature was low while people in the control group were unaffected by weather changes. One point the researchers made was that the amount of pain was not significant enough to predict weather changes.

A conflicting study out of Florida reported a group of patients with osteoarthritis. One hundred and fifty four patients were followed for two years with specific cataloging of daily temperatures, barometric pressures, and precipitation along with symptoms. A slight association of hand pain with rising barometric pressure was found. However, no other significant associations were demonstrated.

Other anecdotal studies have reported that people who live in warmer, drier climates have fewer symptoms than people who live in colder damper climates. An important point: the course of disease is not affected.

So what is to be made of this? I know my patients are very good at predicting imminent weather fronts. In fact, I'll believe them ahead of TV weather people any time. Also, it is apparent to me after many years of experience (I began practice in 1981) that cold damp weather aggravates symptoms.

One old study that seems to make sense was one done by Joseph Hollander at the University of Pennsylvania several years ago. He was able to demonstrate through use of a barometric pressure chamber, that changes in barometric pressure do affect a patient's threshold for feeling arthritis related symptoms. Theorists have suggested that reduction in barometric pressure such as what occurs in cold rainy weather causes expansion of the joint capsule which stretches pain fibers located in the joint leading to pain.

Another possibility is that pain thresholds drop with cold weather. It is also apparent that cloudy damp days affect mood. I've noticed this especially in patients with fibromyalgia and osteoarthritis. Cold weather is also a deterrent to people going outside and getting the needed exercise that helps reduce arthritis pain.

www.arthritistreatmentcenter.com

My own pet theory is that osteoarthritis symptoms are affected by weather changes. Many people with inflammatory forms of arthritis also have osteoarthritis so that symptom flares with weather probably reflect the effect on osteoarthritis.

Weather probably affects inflammatory forms of arthritis less. Warm sunny weather is not a guarantee of improvement in arthritis symptoms. I have numerous rheumatology colleagues who practice in Florida and Arizona and they are very, very busy!

So what advice can I give?

If you are absolutely positive that a warm climate is making your arthritis better and you'd like to move, make sure you spend some time living in the warm area before you actually make the switch. Also realize that when you do make the switch you will be leaving many important components of your support team such as friends, relatives, and physicians behind. This is an important factor to consider.

If you live in a cold area, that shouldn't deter you from living a healthy vigorous lifestyle. Regular exercise can be done indoors as well as it can be done outdoors.

Chapter 19

How do you make the early diagnosis of rheumatoid arthritis?

The cause of the immune abnormality that occurs in rheumatoid arthritis still has no definite explanation. Some suspect an environmental trigger such as a virus or bacterium interacts with specific genes that a patient may have. This leads to a cascade of events culminating in inflammation.

The immune attack occurs at the site of the synovium- the lining of the joints. White blood cells flood this area and release destructive enzymes. This sequence of events leads to inflammation of the synovium, erosion of cartilage and bone, and subsequent weakening of tendons, ligaments, and muscles. Because it is a systemic illness, rheumatoid arthritis may affect other organ systems in the body such as the eyes and heart.

Early diagnosis is not always easy. The joint swelling that is characteristic of rheumatoid arthritis may not be that pronounced. Sometimes fatigue, low-grade fever, weight loss, loss of appetite, and stiffness, may be the chief symptoms- but these symptoms can occur with other diseases as well!

Over a period of a few weeks to months, joint symptoms such as pain, redness, and swelling can develop and be accompanied by loss of function.

Morning stiffness is a key component of rheumatoid arthritis. This generally lasts more than an hour. Patients may also complain of stiffness during the day if they sit for any length of time.

Examination may reveal swelling affecting multiple joints, both small and large- although small joints of the hands, wrists, ankles, and feet are most commonly involved.

Bumps under the skin near joints such as the fingers and elbows may occur. These are called rheumatoid nodules.

Laboratory tests are helpful. Elevation of erythrocyte sedimentation rate (ESR) or C-reactive protein indicates systemic inflammation. A positive rheumatoid factor is seen in about 80-85% of patients. The rheumatoid factor may be negative early on and may be persistently negative in 20% of patients. Anti-CCP- a new diagnostic test – is more specific for rheumatoid arthritis than the rheumatoid factor, which may be positive in other conditions.

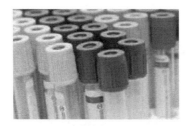

Magnetic resonance imaging (MRI) and diagnostic ultrasound are helpful imaging tests for early diagnosis. X-rays may not become positive until a patient has had their disease for at least six months and are therefore not useful for early diagnosis.

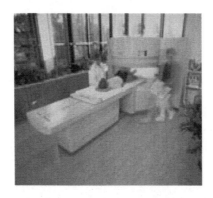

www.arthritistreatmentcenter.com

Chapter 20

Can arthritis kill you?

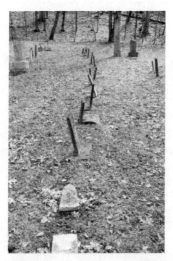

For some time, there has been strong evidence that having rheumatoid arthritis significantly increases one's risk of dying. Mortality data from another recent study seems to confirm the fact that having inflammatory arthritis and then developing cancer is a bad combination. It appears that if one has inflammatory arthritis and develops cancer, then the risk of dying from that cancer is greater than if one did not have inflammatory arthritis.

Patients with rheumatoid arthritis (RA), a chronic inflammatory autoimmune disease, have a high risk of death from disease -- at least double the risk of the general population, studies overwhelmingly show. Evidence has been less clear on whether RA patients are exceptionally vulnerable to dying from cancer.

The first study to investigate whether patients with RA who develop cancer have a decreased rate of survival also examined the impact of rheumatic disease on overall cancer incidence. The study focused on 2,105 patients with recent onset inflammatory polyarthritis (IP). It should be mentioned that over time, a large proportion of new-onset IP cases will evolve into RA.

Researchers in the United Kingdom followed the IP patients over a 10-year period to detect the occurrence of cancer. Among the group, they identified 123 cases of cancer for analysis. These cases included bone, lung, breast, prostate, urinary, colon, and brain cancers; cancers of the digestive, respiratory, and central nervous systems; cancers of the blood cells and cancerous tumors; but excluded non-melanotic skin cancers?

Then, they compared these rates with the rates of cancer in the general population from the same geographic area, adjusting for difference in age and sex.

Overall, the incidence of cancer was not increased in the IP subjects compared with the general population. However, the risk of blood cell cancers was increased among the IP sample, a finding researchers expected given the known association between RA and lymphoma.

The study also compared the number of deaths in patients with cancer and inflammatory arthritis with that of cancer patients without a history of inflammatory arthritis. The finding was striking. There was a 40 percent increase in mortality in patients who suffered both IP or RA, and cancer.

The authors commented that 5-year cancer survival in patients with IP is substantially reduced in comparison with that in the general population, even after adjusting for differences in age, sex, and cancer site, whereas the overall cancer incidence does not seem to be increased.

(Franklin J, Lunt M, Bunn D, Symmons D, Silman A. Influence of Inflammatory Polyarthritis on Cancer Incidence and Survival: Results from a Community-Based Prospective Study. Arthritis Rheum. 2007; 56: 790-798).

Author's note: Statistics regarding the marked increase in mortality from RA are bad enough. This excess mortality appears to be related to the premature atherosclerosis that is seen in RA. However, this recent study really adds more fuel to the fire. Bottom line: RA is not a benign disease and should be treated as a medical emergency.

Chapter 21

How to protect your joints if you have arthritis

If you go a physical or occupational therapist, you will be taught specific ways to protect your joints. Here are a few tips that might help prevent excessive strain on your joints if you suffer from arthritis...

- Pace yourself. You need to balance periods of rest and activity during the day. By managing your workload throughout the day using common sense, you can help avoid overworked joints. Work at a steady, moderate pace and avoid the temptation to be rushed. Plan specific points when you will rest. You should do this before you become fatigued or sore. Alternate light and heavier activities throughout the day. Also, take the time to perform periodic stretch breaks.

- Do not spend too much time in the same position. This causes your joints to become stiff. You must move! For example, if you are watching television, get up and move around every half hour. If you are doing a lot of knitting or writing, take the time every 15-20 minutes to flex your fingers and stretch them. If traveling - take breaks at least once an hour and stretch.

- Forget the old adage, "no pain no gain." If there are activities that cause you to feel sore and achy, stop doing them. There is a difference between the mild tiredness you feel in the muscles when you do something you're unaccustomed to doing and the severe pain that comes from doing something that isn't good for you. Learn to recognize the distinction. Learn to understand and respect your arthritis pain. Any pain lasting longer than an hour after you do the activity means the activity is probably one you should avoid. Perhaps you can modify the activity somehow. You may want to postpone some activities when you are having a severe flare.

- Throughout the day, favor large joints. Use the strongest joint available for the job. Save your smaller joints for the specific jobs that only they can accomplish. As an example, consider carrying objects with your palm open, distributing the weight equally over your forearm instead of the hands and wrists. Using larger muscle groups will reduce stress on small joints. Slide objects along a counter or workbench by pushing them rather than lifting them. Use a loop that you can pull with your wrist or forearm to decrease stress on your fingers if you need to open a cabinet. Don't be afraid to ask for help.

- The hands are the joints that are most easily stressed and subject to injury. You use your fingers in many daily activities. Abnormally stressful positions and techniques can increase the risk of getting deformities. For example, avoid positions that push your other fingers toward your little finger. Finger motions should be in the direction of your thumb whenever possible. This prevents the deviation of the fingers towards the little fingers that is so common in people with rheumatoid arthritis. Here's an example… instead of brushing crumbs off a table with your palm flat on the table, turn your hand so that the little finger is resting on the table and the palm is facing you. Then push the crumbs off the table. This will prevent the fingers from being pushed in the direction of your little finger.

- Another tip: avoid making a tight fist. Use built-up handles on tools and household implements, which will make them easier to hold. By the same token, avoid pinching movements between your thumb and your fingers. For instance, hold a book, plate or mug in the palms of your hands. Use a book holder if you're planning on reading for

www.arthritistreatmentcenter.com

long periods. Instead of a purse with a handle grip, select one with a shoulder strap. Use paper bags instead of plastic bags with handles for groceries.

- The way you carry your body largely affects how much strain you put on your joints. Proper body mechanics allow you to use your body more efficiently and conserve energy. The proper height for a work surface is 2 inches below your bent elbow when you're in the seated position. Make sure you have good back and foot support when you sit. Your forearms and upper legs should be level with the floor.

- If you type at a keyboard for long periods, use a chair with arms. If your chair doesn't have arms, consider using wrist or forearm supports. An angled work surface, like a draftsman's table, is good for reading and writing and is easier on your neck. If you work standing up, the height of your work surface should enable you to work comfortably without having to stoop. Raise the height of your chair. This helps make it easier on your hips and knees as you sit down and get up. If you have to pick up items from the floor stoop by bending your knees and hips. One other trick is to sit in a chair and bend over. Maintain good posture with shoulders back and chin slightly tucked. Pretend that there is a string attached from the top of your head to the ceiling. It will help you stand taller and straighter. Poor posture causes uneven weight distribution and may strain your ligaments and muscles.

- Practice range-of-motion exercises throughout the day. Do these gently.

All of these tips should help you live with less pain and allow you to enjoy life more.

Chapter 22

Part 1: What kinds of exercise can I do if I have arthritis? (indoors)

People with arthritis have pain when they move; so many people with arthritis limit their movement. But this inactivity can be detrimental and lead to more crippling. More than 30 years ago, one of the accepted forms of treatment was bedrest. This was done to help patients with arthritis preserve their joints. It is now recognized that this type of treatment causes more harm than good, in many instances. Studies have revealed that people with arthritis who exercise regularly report less pain and joint swelling, improved functioning and increased strength, endurance and flexibility -- without harming their joints.

The psychological benefits are also important. People who exercise experience less depression and anxiety and greater feelings of control. Confidence in the ability to perform activities of daily living leads to a sense of well-being. There is less fear, particularly when it comes to things like falls. Patients with arthritis often worry about falling and being unable to get back up.

Since people with arthritis range in conditioning from very frail to those who are only slightly limited, the variety of exercises is enormous. There are two major areas to consider: indoor and outdoor.

This article will focus on indoor exercises.

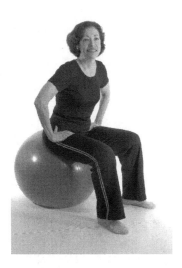

Indoor exercises for people with arthritis fall into three major categories.

1.   Range of motion exercises. These are exercises that help reduce the level of stiffness and keep the joints flexible. The term "range of motion" means the normal distance the joints can move in all directions. There are five primary targets...

- Shoulders. Slow easy arm circles. Starting with arms at the sides, bring them all the way up toward the ceiling and then as far behind the body as comfortable in a huge circle. Repeat 5-10 times.
- Hips. Lie on your back with knees bent, feet on the floor and arms down along the sides. Bring one knee to the chest and rotate the knee in an easy gentle circle. Repeat with other knee. Do this 5-10 times.
- Wrists. Make circles with the wrists, rotating hands in both directions.

www.arthritistreatmentcenter.com

- Ankles. Draw big circles in the air with the big toe in both clockwise and counterclockwise motion.
- Knees. Lie on your back and bring one knee to the chest. Straighten the leg, pointing the foot toward the ceiling and bend a few times. Repeat with the other leg.

2. Non-impact aerobic exercise. People with arthritis need to do 30 minutes a day of cardiovascular activity. In particular, conditioning large muscles, such as those in the legs, stimulates the healing of cartilage. When choosing an exercise, it's important to pick something that doesn't worsen arthritis. Walk on a flat even surface. Here is where indoor and outdoor can mix. For instance, a school track is a good choice. Remember to wear good, comfortable, supportive shoes. If there is no access to a track, consider a mall or a sidewalk. Avoid bumpy fields or gravel roads. Water exercises. For some people, walking is difficult. A good alternative is water exercise. The buoyancy of the water supports the body so there's less stress on the spine, hips and knees. The Arthritis Foundation sometimes sponsors water exercise classes at the YMCA. These classes are good because they allow a person to exercise in water at chest level. They provide good range of motion and aerobic conditioning.

3. Strengthening exercises. There are some excellent studies showing that weight training for people with arthritis is beneficial. Most of these will be done indoors.

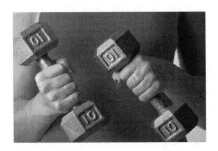

When starting, it's best to begin with light weights such as Heavy Hands or dumbbells and work up from there.

The goal is to work out with a weight that can be lifted at least 10 times without too much effort. If it is too difficult, then the weight is too heavy. Significant injury can result, so be careful! Resistance straps are also an option. Check with your physical therapist. Here are some good lower body strengthening exercises.

- Leg extensions. Sit straight in a chair, knees bent 90 degrees, feet flat on floor. Then extend the leg straight out, hold it for 10 seconds, then bend it back down to the starting position. Start with 10 to 15 repetitions and increase to 50 over time.
- Toe raises. Work the calves by standing and raising the body up on tiptoes and back down. Do 8 to 10 repetitions.
- Chair squats. Sit in a chair and practice standing straight up and sitting back down again, using the muscles of the legs. It strengthens the legs and also helps with balance.

Always check with your rheumatologist before starting this or any other exercise program.

Chapter 23

Part 2: What kinds of exercise can I do if I have arthritis? (outdoors)

Outdoor exercises are obviously more rigorous. An earlier chapter discussed indoor exercises.

The type of outdoor exercise a person can engage in if they have arthritis is definitely a function of their motivation, training, and interest.

For instance, my son has juvenile ankylosing spondylitis yet played varsity soccer in high school. One of my sisters has had severe rheumatoid arthritis for more than 20 years and runs marathons.

Now I'm not suggesting that these are the types of outdoor exercises that all people with arthritis should engage in. However, I am mentioning these two examples to show readers what is possible.

Hiking is a very good form of exercise. Make sure to wear comfortable shoes that provide ankle support. Get a trail map and get going! If one is a novice, it's best to start on less hilly terrain. Once conditioning has improved, then hills can enter into the equation.

One outdoor activity that is growing in popularity is kayaking. Kayaking involves using a paddle to propel a boat in a continuous motion. Kayaking is a low-impact sport so there are no injuries from pounding, and it can be done at a pace that suits the individual. It is particularly good for strengthening back and upper body muscles. This helps improve posture. Since it is an enjoyable activity that is done outdoors against the backdrop of nature, people benefit from fresh air, a change of scenery, as well as exercise. An instructor can teach the best method for getting upright if one should capsize. And always wear a life jacket. For more comfort, select a boat that has back support and bring along kneepads or washcloths to put between the knees and the boat's hard front edge.

A similar exercise is rowing. In fact, rowing is probably one of the more aerobic types of exercise. However, people with low back problems or knee problems might want to avoid this.

Another popular hobby is gardening. Gardening is great for increased flexibility and stretching. A person can garden by themselves and enjoy solitude or enjoy the camaraderie of a community garden or gardening club.

Winter provides a number of outdoor opportunities. Snowshoeing is one of the best forms of exercise available. There are a variety of types, and they all fit easily onto hiking boots. Snowshoe technology has made it so easy that walking on snow is almost identical to hiking.

Skiing and even snowboarding are activities that the more adventurous and more in shape adult can enjoy. Obviously, both of these activities are at the top of the scale in terms of difficulty for people with arthritis. However, very few activities outdoors are as much fun once they are mastered. Cross country skiing is less difficult to master than downhill and is an excellent form of aerobic exercise.

Skating, of course, is another good cold weather exercise. Previous experience is a plus. Make sure that a helmet is worn and the skates are a good fit. Also make sure that balance is not a big issue as it might be with people who take certain medications such as high blood pressure drugs. Skating is actually a good way to improve balance.

Another outdoor activity for older adults is bicycling. Biking is easy on the joints. It is aerobic, strengthening and lots of fun. What if it's raining cats and dogs or there's a blizzard? Ballroom dancing and tap dancing are becoming favorites with many adults. Dancing is aerobic and weight bearing, so it's good for the bones. Most communities have a nearby dance school. It's also a great social outlet.

Always check with your rheumatologist before starting this or any exercise program.

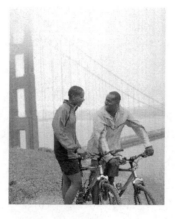

Chapter 24

Doctor, what's the best type of exercise for arthritis?

Patients with arthritis benefit from exercise. Numerous studies have documented the improvement in strength and endurance that people with arthritis have who regularly engage in exercise versus those that don't.

A good exercise program combines elements of aerobic, strengthening, and stretching. So what is the single best type of exercise? The answer is "all wet."

Water exercise appears to be the single best form of exercise for people with arthritis. The buoyancy of the water relieves stress on joints. Because of buoyancy, people with arthritis can improve flexibility, perform movements, and even do strength training without the impact these exercises would have on the joints on land. The water temperature should be warm. The warmth creates a soothing environment for painful joints. The warmth also relaxes muscles and improves blood flow.

It's important to get medical clearance from your physician before embarking on any kind of exercise program. A physical therapist can help design a good water exercise program for you.

Spend at least 10-15 minutes warming up and stretching before starting your exercise program.

Doing water exercise at least 3-4 times per week is best. Each session should last about 30 minutes or so.

Make sure you move the joints gently without sudden jerking movements. Go through a full range of motion.

Start slowly. This isn't a race. You can build endurance over time. As your fitness improves, you can consider other forms of water exercise such as jogging with a buoyancy vest, using water resistance paddles, and lap swimming, etc. Always make sure a lifeguard is present.

Water exercise can also supplement a land exercise program.

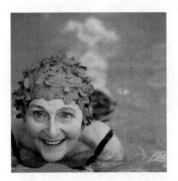

Chapter 25

I have arthritis – how do I lose weight?

Patients with arthritis, particularly osteoarthritis (OA), need to maintain weight at an ideal level. Ideal body weight is dependent on what your body mass index (BMI) is. There are charts available that can tell you what your BMI is.

> Weight categories: BMI
> Underweight <18.5
> Normal 18.5-24.9
> Overweight 25-29.9
> Obese >30

Why is weight so important for arthritis? Studies have shown that overweight or obese women who lose about 11 pounds (2 BMI units) decrease the risk of having OA of the knees by 50 percent. Gaining 11 pounds increases the risk of knee OA by 28 percent.

While the correlation with symptoms is still uncertain, it seems clear that there is added stress on the body with excess weight.

For instance the force exerted on the hip and knee during walking is about three times one's body weight. Overweight and obese people could conceivably be increasing damage to cartilage. Alteration of gait -the way one walks- would also have detrimental effects on the weight bearing joints. Obese people do tend to alter their gait.

Some evidence suggests that obese people also have circulating hormones and growth factors that also could aggravate the development of OA.

Weight loss is simple... but not easy. Essentially you have to take in fewer calories than you use up. That means a combination of diet and exercise is what is required.

It may be as simple as avoiding high fat snacks and limiting portion size. Men over the age of 50 should reduce caloric intake to 1,800 calories a day while women over the age of 50 should limit their caloric intake to less than 1,400 calories a day. If this is combined with a moderate exercise program, weight should come off at a rate of 1 to 2 pounds a week.

Limit activities such as TV watching...

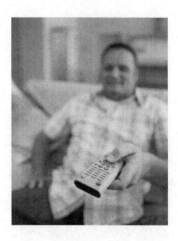

Exercise is key. Exercise not only helps with weight control but it can also strengthen the muscles that protect joints. You should start slow but aim for 30 to 40 minutes 6 days a week as an eventual goal.

Aerobic exercise such as walking, riding a stationary bike, using an elliptical trainer or cross country ski machine may all be helpful. Swimming is another great form of exercise as is a rowing machine. (Avoid using a rower if you have low back problems.)

www.arthritistreatmentcenter.com

Weight training is helpful. And stretching should also be considered as an important component of any exercise program. Tai chi is a useful form of exercise for some people.

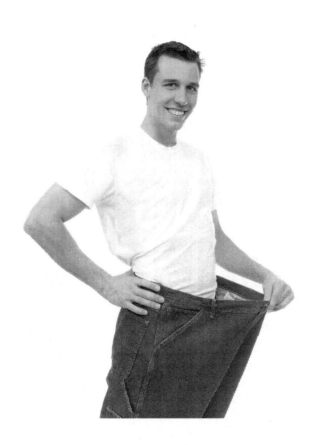

Chapter 26

Consumer tips regarding nutritional supplements for people with arthritis

Today, more than ever, dietary supplements are being sold and being consumed by patients with arthritis. Unfortunately, many people don't know how to read a dietary supplement label. This chapter discusses how to do that.

Knowing how to take nutritional supplements is exceedingly important for anyone but especially important for patients with arthritis who are already taking a number of other medicines. Here are important tips to know. Safety first: Know what you are taking, what it is used for, and how much to take. Dietary supplements may interact with prescription and over the counter as well as other supplements and foods.

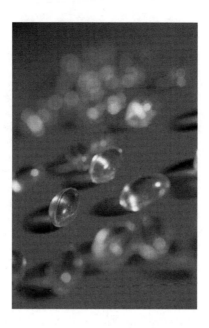

Always read the label and look for warnings, cautions, interactions, or side effects. Talk to your doctor or pharmacist about all medications and dietary supplements you take. Never take dietary supplements instead of prescribed drugs unless you first talk with your doctor.

Remember, dietary supplements are not meant to treat or cure diseases. Do not believe the hype. If a product sounds too good to be true, it probably is. No product can treat a wide range of unrelated ailments or health conditions.

Learn all you can about the products before you take them. Natural doesn't always mean safe. Natural products, while not synthesized chemically, may still have the same side effects as similar products produced in a laboratory. Look for reputable companies. These companies will provide contact information to receive more product information or answer questions or complaints. If you have any questions or concerns about a product, call or write to the company. If the company does not respond, do not use the product.

www.arthritistreatmentcenter.com

Chapter 27

Which oil supplements work for rheumatoid arthritis... and which don't!

"Your food shall be your remedy. Let food be your medicine and let medicine be your food..."

These words were uttered by Hippocrates.

With all the emphasis on natural remedies currently, one area of great interest is the use of food-based oils to help with different disease processes, particularly arthritis.

Most American diets are high in oils called omega-6 fatty acids (linoleic acid) which eventually are broken down to arachodonic acid, which is a cornerstone of inflammation...obviously, not something that is desirable.

So if that's the bad oil, what are the good ones?

One good oil is omega-3 which helps to reduce inflammation. Another good fatty acid is gamma linoleic acid or GLA. So... to get the best effect, one should try to reduce the amount of omega 6 and increase the amount of both omega-3 and gamma linoleic acid.

Fish oil is the source of omega-3 fatty acid that has been studied most carefully. Numerous studies have demonstrated its effectiveness in reducing the risk of cardiovascular events as well as reducing the inflammation that accompanies rheumatoid arthritis (RA). Fish oil is available as both a liquid or as a softgel capsule. The typical daily dose is 3 grams per day of EPA/DHA, the active ingredients in fish oil.

If you would like to get your dose of fish oil naturally, you can eat the following types of fish: salmon, tuna, sardines, herring, and mackerel. Omega-3 is abundant in cold water fish.

Another good oil that contains high amounts of GLA is evening primrose oil. Another good source of GLA is borage seed oil. These preparations have been shown to help with the symptoms of RA. Dosage for RA is 1.8 grams of GLA per day.

Another oil that increases the amounts of EPA is flaxseed oil. Flaxseed oil can be used in salad dressings. Flaxseed flour can be used to make baked products.

When purchasing products it's important to read the labels carefully. The packaging should be in opaque containers. Try to get high potency capsules.

Also, be wary of potential side effects. Fish oil and GLA can thin the blood. This is particularly a problem in patients who are taking nonsteroidal anti-inflammatory drugs (NSAIDS), blood thinners like Coumadin, or other herbal remedies such as ginger which can thin the blood also.

Be patient. It takes at least three months before you will notice a benefit.

Some patients do develop gastrointestinal side effects such as gas or heartburn. Also, burps will have a fishy smell. Fish oil can also be excreted with sweat so that you may smell like the local seafood market.

Do not use these oils as your only therapy for RA. It's important to realize that these oils are complementary (used in addition to) conventional medications.

In addition to the above advice, try lowering the amount red meat you eat. Red meat is high in ingredients that promote the inflammatory process.

One word of caution. Because omega-3 supplements are available without prescription, they are not covered by insurance... so beware.

Chapter 28

Some foods make my arthritis worse... is it my imagination?

While conventional treatments for rheumatoid arthritis (RA) are extremely effective in most instances, they do present problems in regards to safety. In recent years, a resurgent interest in the use of alternative therapies has been noted. The response to these treatments is variable and many times unpredictable. However, some patients have had dramatic improvement or even complete remission. This observation makes alternative therapies worth looking at. For centuries, the effects of food on arthritis symptoms have been discussed both in the scientific literature as well as in lay writings. Food allergy has been reported to play a role particularly in RA.

In a study published in 1980, 22 patients with RA consumed a diet that excluded common allergens. Twenty patients (91%) experienced an improvement in symptoms, and 19 found that specific foods repeatedly exacerbated their symptoms. The mean time on the elimination diet before improvement occurred was 10 days, and the longest time was 18 days. The mean number of food sensitivities per patient was 2.5; the most common symptom-provoking foods were grains, milk, nuts, beef, and egg. (Hicklin JA, McEwen LM, Morgan JE. The effect of diet in rheumatoid arthritis. Clin Allergy 1980;10:463.)

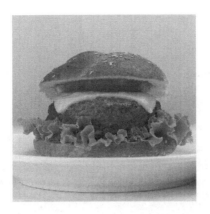

In a later study, 53 patients with RA were randomly assigned to consume a diet that excluded common allergens, or their usual diet (control group) for six weeks. After one week, the patients on the exclusion diet began reintroducing one food at a time; any foods producing symptoms were removed from the diet. The hypoallergenic diet group faired significantly better than the control group for each of 13 different parameters of disease activity. The patients in the control group then underwent the same elimination and challenge procedure that the diet group had, and experienced similar, though somewhat less impressive, improvements (Darlington LG, Ramsey NW, Mansfield JR. Placebo-controlled, blind study of dietary manipulation therapy in rheumatoid arthritis. Lancet 1986;1:236-238).

Long-term follow-up of 100 patients who underwent dietary therapy in this study revealed that one-third remained well on diet alone, without any medication, for up to 7.5 years after starting treatment (Darlington LG, Ramsey NW. Diets for rheumatoid arthritis. Lancet 1991;338:1209).

While the possibility of placebo effect needs to be considered, the long term benefit experienced by these patients is noteworthy. Also, while there was some weight loss noted in the treated patients, there was no significant correlation between weight loss and clinical improvement in RA symptoms.

In another double-blind controlled study, 94 patients with RA were randomized to one of two diets for four weeks, followed by a return to their usual diets for another four weeks.

One diet ("allergen free") was free of common allergens, additives and preservatives. The other diet ("low allergen") was similar to the allergen-free diet, but contained milk allergens and azo dyes. Seventy-eight patients completed the study. The effects of food elimination and re-challenge varied considerably among patients. Nine patients (11.5% of the total; 6 in the allergen-free group, 3 in the low-allergen group) had a favorable response to the elimination diet, followed by marked disease flare during re-challenge. In these patients, subjective improvements were confirmed by improvements in objective parameters of disease activity (Van de Laar MA, van der Korst JK. Food intolerance in rheumatoid arthritis. I. A double blind, controlled trial of the clinical effects of elimination of milk allergens and azo dyes. Ann Rheum Dis 1992;51:298-302).

The small number of patients exhibiting changes is an argument against significant benefits associated with a diet manipulation. Nonetheless it appears that there is a subset of patients for whom diet is an important component of their symptom complex.

A smaller study looked at eleven RA patients. Two of the 11 RA patients showed a favorable response to an elimination diet and experienced worsening after eating offending foods. In that study, the elimination diet did not exclude certain common allergens (wheat, corn, egg whites, sugar, and coffee). It could be argued that the response rate would have been higher if the elimination diet had been more restrictive (Panush RS, Carter RL, Katz P, et al. Diet therapy for rheumatoid arthritis. Arthritis Rheum 1983;26:462-471). Small numbers in this study make comprehensive validation impossible.

These studies seem to imply that avoidance of allergenic foods might benefit a subset of patients with RA, although the proportion of patients responding to dietary change varies a lot from one study to the next. The difference in response rates may be related in part to the patient populations studied. Some authorities feel that younger patients (under the age of 40) with less aggressive RA respond best to avoidance of allergens. Older patients and those with relatively severe RA may not respond to dietary manipulation as well. The divergent results in published studies may also be explained in part by strictness of dietary restriction and/or compliance. Finally, RA is a spectrum of diseases; not all therapies work for all patients. This divergence of effect has been noted even with biologic therapies.

The possibility of food allergies accounting for RA symptoms makes the use of food allergy testing a viable weapon in the arsenal of the clinical rheumatologist. In our clinic we use food allergy testing in patients where symptoms don't seem to respond to conventional therapies.

Chapter 29

Seven insider food secrets that help you beat arthritis... by an arthritis expert

The term "arthritis" is derived from the Greek... "arthron" meaning joint... and "itis" meaning inflammation. Most types of arthritis are associated with inflammation. Inflammation is a defense mechanism the body employs to fight infection, tumors, and other foreign invaders. The mediator of this inflammatory response is the immune system.

Picture an army of warriors – the immune response- which is ready and eager to take on the task of protecting you against enemies. Inflammation is regulated so that under normal circumstances, once the problem is taken care of, inflammation stops. Unfortunately, inflammation can escape this control mechanism and become chronic. Chronic inflammation, it is believed, is the underlying basis for the development of diseases such as arthritis, diabetes, and heart disease.

So is there a way to manipulate the diet so that arthritis damage caused by inappropriate inflammation can be controlled? Recent research has suggested that diets that contain omega-3 fatty acids that combat inflammation may be useful. Also, the elimination of foods containing omega-6 fatty acids which promote inflammation is also helpful.

Here is a list of seven "insider secrets" that you should know about.

Secret #1:   Make cold water fish part of your diet at least two to three times a week. Examples include cold water salmon (not farm raised), sardines, herring, cod, and trout. The reason? These types of fish are rich in omega-3 fatty acids. If fish is something you don't enjoy, consider flax seed, walnuts, or dietary fish supplements… all of which also contain significant amounts of omega-3. (Note: If you are a blood thinner, consult your doctor before taking a dietary supplements with omega-3 since your drug dose may need to be adjusted.)

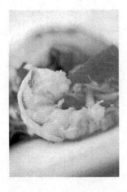

Secret #2:   Reduce the amount of certain oils such as corn oil, sunflower oil, and safflower oil. These contain large amounts of omega-6 fatty acids that promote inflammation. Use olive oil or canola oil instead.

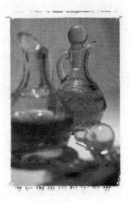

www.arthritistreatmentcenter.com

Secret # 3:   Go for veggies and fruits. Many vegetables and fruits are high in antioxidants that fight inflammation. Berries such as blueberries and cherries are excellent and tasty sources of anti-inflammatory ingredients. Pineapple is a good source of bromelain, an excellent antioxidant.

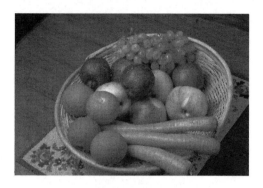

Secret # 4:   Avoid the white poisons. Often ingredients like refined sugar, refined flour and salt are used in the production of processed foods such as white bread, sugary cereals, candies, and pastries. These white poisons promote inflammation and should be avoided.

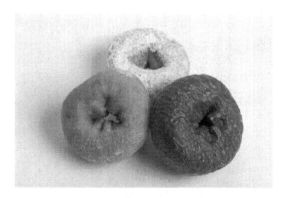

Secret # 5:   Reduce the amount of red meat in your diet: Animal
                protein contains large amounts of pro-inflammatory
                fatty acids.

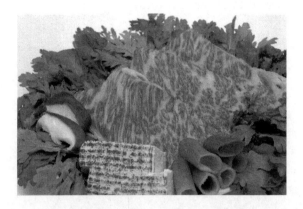

Secret #6:   Reduce the amount of trans fat in your diet. Trans fats,
                which are present in fried foods, cakes, pies, cookies,
                and other baked goods, increase low density cholesterol
                (LDL). This is the bad cholesterol that is pro-
                inflammatory.

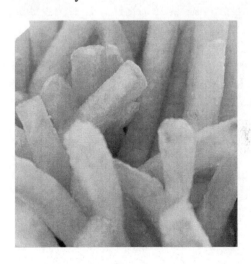

Secret # 7:   Use more spices: Spices such as curcumin, garlic, and ginger, contain ingredients which have been shown in some well-controlled studies to reduce the inflammation of arthritis.

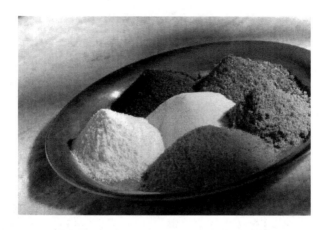

Some people have claimed that dairy products and nightshade vegetables such as eggplant, potatoes, and tomatoes, cause their arthritis to get worse. There may be some individual food sensitivities/ allergies that do aggravate arthritis. However, a blanket statement about the role of dairy products and nightshade plants is not warranted. At our center we do suggest the use of food allergy testing in individuals who have arthritic symptoms that are troublesome and appear to be food-induced. For more information about food allergy testing, call us at (301) 694-5800.

Finally, dietary manipulation should not be used as a substitute for proper and aggressive conventional medical care. A rheumatologist should be consulted.

Chapter 30

How do I get arthritis pain relief?

Arthritis pain relief starts with knowing when to rest and when not to. In the example of a person with osteoarthritis of the knee for example, it has been demonstrated that regular exercise is essential to maintaining strength and flexibility as well as controlling pain.

On the flip side, overdoing exercise can lead to increased pain. So... the lesson here is that activity and exercise should be increased slowly with medical supervision.

Assistive devices such as corrective shoes, canes, braces, heel wedges or other inserts may reduce pain and delay the need for knee replacement surgery.

Over-the-counter analgesics (acetaminophen) or anti-inflammatory drugs (ibuprofen, naproxyn) are also helpful. Potential side effects such as liver and kidney dysfunction and stomach ulcers must be taken into consideration.

Topical remedies such as capsaicin containing creams may also provide temporary relief. A new topical agent called MyoRx contains omega-3 fatty acids which are anti-inflammatory and may be superior to capsaicin creams.

Heat and cold are helpful. Moist heat is effective for muscle spasm related pain and for situations where inflammation is not a major problem. When inflammation is evident, ice makes more sense. Care must be taken to limit the exposure to either heat or ice to no more than 20 minutes at a time.

For supporting and protecting inflamed joints, splints and braces often are very effective. Use of splints and braces should be used in concert with anti-inflammatory medicine, injections, and physical therapy to prevent the development of loss of joint mobility.

Assistive devices for home use may make activities such as opening jars, turning faucets, reaching for items on the floor much easier and less painful.

Weight loss in patients with osteoarthritis of weight bearing regions such as the low back, hips, and knees is mandatory for heavy people.

Cortisone injections can provide pain relief when other measures are insufficient. Injections of hyaluronic acid which is a lubricant may also be effective.

Supplements such as glucosamine/chondroitin (one of the best is Joint Food) and omega-3 oils (a pure form is Sea Gold) can be helpful. Information about MyoRx, Joint Food, and Sea Gold is available at www.arthritistreatmentcenter.com .

Oral anti-inflammatory medicines and narcotic analgesics may also be required. These should be given by physicians who are skilled in using these drugs.

A transcutaneous nerve stimulator (TENS) unit also is worth a try for people with chronic pain issues. This is a device that a patient wears clipped to their belt. The device is attached to a sticky electrode that adheres to the skin. The TENS produces a small electric current and blocks pain impulses that travel over peripheral nerves.

Chapter 31

Doctor ...I'm afraid of drugs... What alternative or complementary therapies seem to work?

Complementary therapies- also called alternative therapies- are gaining more popularity because of the fear that many people have of pharmaceutical products.

Many of these complementary treatments are common sense measures that depend on lifestyle changes. Alterations in diet, institution of exercise programs, cessation of tobacco, reduction in alcohol consumption, control of stress are considered to fall under the "complementary" umbrella but have been advocated for many years by traditional physicians as well.

Complementary therapies should not necessarily be used exclusively. The word "complementary" indicates that these therapies should be used alongside traditional medicines. And it is that combination- traditional plus complementary- that seems to offer the best long term results.

One of the leaders in both traditional as well as complementary medicine approaches has been the venerable Mayo Clinic. The director of the Mayo Complementary and Integrative Medicine Division, Dr. Amit Sood, has listed the major criteria that they use to determine the suitability of a complementary approach.

Safety. This is vitally important because if this therapy does no harm it is generally worth trying. While it may not be effective, there is no harm in trying it.

- Fills a void. Conventional medicines sometimes don't address key issues of importance. An example is stress. The traditional approach has been to use mood stabilizers or other similar drugs. These drugs have undesirable side effects in many instances. That makes the institution of complementary approaches such as meditation, guided imagery, yoga, and tai chi more attractive.
- Standardization. This is a biggie because there is very little regulation of the nutritional supplement industry. What is on the label is not necessarily what you get. The best defense is to either buy from a reputable company (and even this isn't a guarantee!) or ask a knowledgeable physician.
- Does it help people other than the patient? People who are constantly around the patient, e.g. relatives and friends can also benefit from certain complementary therapies. An example is music therapy… although if the patient is an aficionado of rap and his father is not, this may not necessarily work!

So what are some of the complementary approaches that seem to work for arthritis?

Let's start with nutritional supplements and herbs. A new term for the use of supplements is to refer to them as "nutriceuticals."

Glucosamine sulfate and chondroitin have been shown to be effective for osteoarthritis in a number of clinical trials. While there have also been some negative studies as well, the preponderance of proof still favors efficacy.

Omega-3 fish oil has also been demonstrated to have a salutai in rheumatoid arthritis. SamE and MSM are supplements with good data. Other herbal products that have shown some anti-inflammatory effects include flaxseed oil, boswellia, black currant oil, bromelain, turmeric (curcumin), borage oil, vitamins C, E, A, D, trace minerals (selenium, boron, calcium, copper), Coenzyme Q10, plant-based compounds (lutein, Cat's claw, capsaicin, quercitin, acidophilis, green tea, grape seed, gotu, bilberry, garlic, Phellodendron Amurense, Phytodolor , stinging nettle, thundergod vine, willow bark).

The Mayo Clinic's picks for the ten best are:

1. Acupuncture. Acupuncture is an ancient Chinese medical treatment. The theory is that life force, chi, travels along well-defined channels called meridians. Placing acupuncture needles at specific spots can alter energy flow. Mayo Clinic opines... "Acupuncture can ...relieve many types of pain, including that from osteoarthritis, low back pain, neck pain..." One large German study of 3,000 patients with hip or knee osteoarthritis found that those receiving acupuncture had more pain relief than those who did not. Other studies looking at acupuncture in osteoarthritis have been inconclusive. Some authorities feel the benefit may be placebo or expectation related. A closely related art is acupressure where manual pressure substitutes for needle insertion.

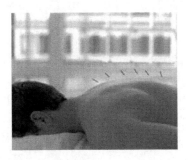

2.   Guided imagery. Also called visualization, this treatment involves using the mind to conjure up visions of an enjoyable soothing environment such as a beach or a mountain lake, etc.

The Mayo people say, "Guided imagery helps reduce anxiety in patients who become claustrophobic during magnetic resonance imaging (MRI) scans, who are having outpatient surgery without general anesthesia or who have been diagnosed with a life-threatening disease, such as cancer." In arthritis, guided imagery is one of the techniques that is employed in cognitive behavioral therapy which is a particularly useful treatment modality for fibromyalgia.

3.   Hypnosis. Either self-hypnosis or formal hypnosis by a therapist can be very effective for dealing with chronic disease and chronic pain.

4.   Massage. Massage has been used to treat lower back pain. It also is effective for fibromyalgia. People with chronic neck and low back problems definitely find this to be helpful.

5.   Meditation. Breathing techniques coupled with the use of a word, called a mantra, which is chanted during the breathing has a beneficial effect on anxiety and stress.

6.   Music therapy. This is a very commonly used therapy. Listening to Baroque or other types of classical music has a calming influence and has been used to treat patients suffering from a variety of chronic illnesses.

7.   Spinal manipulation. This therapy is performed by chiropractors, osteopaths and physical therapists. Mayo writes, "Spinal manipulation is an accepted medical

practice for low back pain, but the evidence supporting its use for other medical problems has been somewhat conflicting."

The UCLA School of Public Health did a study that found chiropractic care as useful as traditional medical care (including the use of painkilling drugs), in relieving discomfort. Other studies have demonstrated that chiropractic is particularly useful for acute painful low back conditions. (A note of caution: patients with osteoporosis should exercise care before undergoing spinal manipulation).

For sure, though, the disdain that used to be shown by traditional medicine for chiropractic no longer should exist.

8.   Spirituality. While belief in a higher being is almost universal, the use of prayer as a therapy has only recently been accepted by traditional medicine. In a number of studies, researchers have demonstrated not only beneficial clinical responses but have also, in some instances, shown actual changes in cellular immune function as a result of prayer. In a least one study, rheumatoid arthritis symptoms improved significantly with prayer.

9.   Tai chi. This is a gentle exercise that has its roots in ancient Chinese tradition. It involves a series of postures and movements performed slowly and gracefully. It is recommended to improve balance in older people to prevent their falling. A study conducted in the Netherlands found those who practiced tai chi had 50 percent fewer falls and fewer injury-causing falls than those who did not.

10.   Yoga. This discipline incorporates stretching and breathing exercises. Originally, an Indian discipline, it has been

found to be effective for relief of stress, lower back pain, carpal tunnel syndrome, and osteoarthritis.

There are some glaring omissions in the Mayo list. I have already discussed nutritional supplements above. Another omission is ultra high frequency electrical stimulation. This modality is actually a mainstream therapy that uses high frequency electrical impulses to depolarize nerve fibers and induce muscle relaxation. This is very useful for chronic neck and low back pain.

Another modality that is gaining more appreciation for its effectiveness in chronic pain is low level laser. Also known as cold laser, this is a gentle easily administered form of light energy that works quite well for chronic neck and low back pain as well as fibromyalgia.

Chapter 32

What herbal remedies can I use for my arthritis?

There are a number of non-medicine treatments to consider for arthritis. The goals of arthritis treatment, regardless of treatment chosen, are to reduce pain, improve mobility, reduce the likelihood of side effects, and enhance the quality of life.

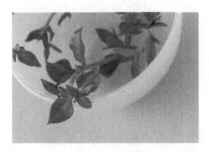

Berries including cherries and blueberries are packed with proanthocyanidins and anthocyanidins. These compounds act as potent antioxidants.

Cayenne pepper is often incorporated into arthritis creams and rubs. It acts on substance P, a chemical neurotransmitter found in nerves. It is helpful for reducing the pain of osteoarthritis.

Celery seed extract has mild anti-inflammatory properties.

Curcumin, also known as turmeric, is a spice that is used in South Asian cooking. It has potent anti-inflammatory effects.

www.arthritistreatmentcenter.com

Devil's claw is an herb that can be found in many health food stores. It has been shown to have analgesic and anti-inflammatory properties.

Fish oil contains omega-3 fatty acids. These are anti-inflammatory and beneficial for people who have rheumatoid arthritis.

Flaxseed also contains omega-3 fatty acids. The concentration is lower than it is in fish oil.

Ginger root has analgesic and anti-inflammatory properties.

Horsetail has beneficial effects (though not entirely proven) on connective tissue. It is touted as a substance that may enhance the strength of tendons and cartilage.

Licorice root has anti-inflammatory effects. It should be used with caution by people who have hypertension because it can elevate blood pressure and cause loss of potassium in the urine.

White willow bark is where aspirin was first discovered. It has analgesic and anti-inflammatory effects.

Yucca root has been used by some for its analgesic effects in arthritis.

With all these herbal remedies, it is important to let your rheumatologist know about them so dosage adjustments in your prescription drugs can be made if necessary.

Chapter 33

Tell me about folk cures for arthritis...

Arthritis is a term that is derived from the Greek... "arthron" for joint, and "itis" for inflammation. It is used to refer to more than 100 different conditions.

It affects almost 70 million Americans and that is the source of folk remedies. Since arthritis is so common and so many people have tried different types of treatments, there are some remedies that are passed on from generation to generation. This goes on despite the lack of supporting medical evidence that prove they actually do work. Rarely though, these remedies have been found- through scientific scrutiny- to have anti-inflammatory properties.

The popular radio announcer Paul Harvey mentioned gin-soaked raisins in the 1990's. This became an overnight arthritis treatment sensation.

Although the formula varies slightly according to what person you talk to, the basics are simple: Eat nine gin-soaked raisins a day. Is there a possible scientific explanation? In this case, there may be. Resveratrol is a bioflavenoid- a powerful antioxidant- that is present in the skin of grapes. Could it be this fact that explains the effectiveness of this age-old remedy? *Gin soaked raisins: Take a box of golden raisins (these are sometimes called white raisins); place in shallow container; cover raisins with distilled gin; let soak for a few weeks until gin evaporates; place in jar; eat nine raisins a day.*

Bee stings: There is scientific evidence that bee venom may contain potent anti-inflammatory ingredients. It is very important not to try this on your own. Also, if you are allergic to bee stings, definitely do not do this. *Apple cider vinegar: Two tablespoons of apple cider vinegar in 8 ounces of water, three times a day. Some people sweeten with honey or add baking soda for pH balance. There is a preparation sold in our area called "Jogging in a Jug". It is a mixture of vinegar and grape juice. Some of my patients swear it helps them.*

Eat spicy foods: There is actually proof with this. Foods containing garlic, ginger, capsaicin, curcumin, and the like do have anti-inflammatory properties.

Avoid tomatoes and other nightshade vegetables: This is a gray area. Some people do seem to have a problem with certain foods causing their arthritis to flare. This is an area of some interest in that food allergy may play a role. The jury is still out.

Gelatin: You can buy gelatin capsules or you can make gelatin (the store variety like Jell-O) but instead of chilling it, drink it. Some suggest drinking a cup a week; you can drink more if you wish. Some people make potions with grape juice and pectin (a jam thickener, such as *Certo*, that contains gelatin powders).

Fresh Pineapple: Eat fresh pineapple frequently for the bromelain, an enzyme found in fresh pineapple (freezing or canning is thought to destroy the enzymes so eat fresh). Bromelain can also be purchased in capsule form as a supplement.

Copper Bracelet: Some believe that copper is absorbed by the skin to relieve joint pain when wearing a copper bracelet but the results are anecdotal and effects controversial. If you wear one, pay a little extra for ones with anti-tarnish coating.

Magnets: Static magnet therapy is believed to relieve pain by increasing circulation, but that has not been proven through numerous scientific studies. Magnetic treatment is considered harmless unless it squeezes your pocketbook too hard.

Rub WD-40 on a joint: I don't know how many times I've heard this one. There is no scientific or otherwise proof this works.

The bottom line to all of these remedies is this: the user should use common sense and his or her own research including consultation with a rheumatologist.

Chapter 34

Doctor... does acupuncture work for arthritis?

Traditional Chinese medicine has used acupuncture to relieve pain as well as to cure disease. During an acupuncture session, a practitioner will insert thin needles into the skin at any one of more than 2,000 carefully defined meridian points. The ancient theory of why acupuncture is effective is that needle insertion restores qi (life force) flow throughout the channels of the body. When qi is at optimal levels, there is harmony with the universal forces of yin and yang. This leads to improved health and relief of pain.

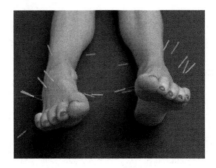

While the traditional acupuncture approach has been to use the needles by themselves, modern acupuncturists may rotate the needles or apply low levels of electric current to improve the effectiveness of the procedure. Sometimes acupressure is also given during the same session. Moxibustion which is the use of herbs that are burned during the procedure is also used. Some practitioners also use "cupping" which is a method where suction cups are applied to meridian points.

Theories as to how acupuncture relieves pain have included the "gate theory" which suggests that pain signals travel along neural pathways through "gates." If a competing stimulus such as acupuncture needles, then pain signals are blocked.

Another theory has to do with endorphin release by the brain due to acupuncture stimulus. Another theory is that acupuncture helps produce analgesic neurotransmitters in the spinal cord.

One large study of acupuncture in osteoarthritis of the knee was performed at the University of Maryland. Researchers compared traditional Chinese acupuncture with sham acupuncture (using either retractable needles or real needles inserted into false pressure points). The study group consisted of 570 patients who reported limited benefits from anti-inflammatory medication and exercise.

The study demonstrated a statistically significant improvement in both pain measures as well as mobility measures in patients receiving real acupuncture versus sham acupuncture.

The authors concluded that "True traditional Chinese acupuncture is safe and effective for reducing pain and improving function in patients with symptomatic knee osteoarthritis who have moderate or greater pain despite background therapy."

Some notes of caution. The effect of acupuncture in relieving pain is not huge. The effects are modest and do take time. The second issue is that the placebo effect undoubtedly enters into the equation.

An interesting study from Dr. George Lewith in Southampton, England used positron emission technology to demonstrate that brain blood flow was altered in a different manner with real acupuncture compared with sham acupuncture therefore validating the concept of a real pain modulating effect of acupuncture on the brain.

Unfortunately, acupuncture does take a long time to work. Dr. Hochberg from the University of Maryland states, "You really have to give acupuncture... six months in order to get maximum benefits from it."

Another downside is the cost. Generally, the charge is anywhere from 60 to 100 dollars a session. Expect that it will cost about $2,000.00. Fortunately, some insurance carriers will cover the cost.

Acupuncture will not be a substitute for conventional treatment. You should use it in conjunction with your regular arthritis therapy. Make sure you see a licensed practitioner.

Chapter 35

What are the risks to my stomach if I take arthritis pain relievers?

The furor over the use of nonsteroidal anti-inflammatory drugs and the relationship to heart disease has overshadowed a more common potential area of toxicity- the gastrointestinal system. This article discusses the risk.

Non-steroidal anti-inflammatory drugs (NSAIDS) are useful for the relief of acute and chronic pain. Patients with both osteoarthritis and rheumatoid arthritis are often treated with these medicines. A significant problem associated with these drugs is the effects on the stomach and bowel.

In particular, adverse effects are noted on the lining of the gut- the gastrointestinal mucosa.

This side effect can present in a number of ways including: esophagitis (inflammation of the esophagus); esophageal stricture (narrowing of the esophagus); gastritis (inflammation of the stomach lining); mucosal erosions (holes in the protective lining of the bowel wall); bleeding; as well as the development of ulcers in the stomach or duodenum (beginning of the small intestine) or its complications including perforation, bowel obstruction, and death.

Also, the small and large bowel mucosa can be affected leading to narrowing of the bowel. This is called a stricture and can lead to bowel obstruction. There is also evidence that NSAIDS can affect the permeability of the gut, possibly allowing the development of antigen antibody reactions to occur. This is the basis for the theories regarding food allergies.

www.arthritistreatmentcenter.com

Although patients may develop important NSAID-caused GI damage with no warning, the following are known risk factors for the development of GI toxicity associated with NSAIDs:

- Age greater than 65 years
- History of peptic ulcer disease or bleeding from the GI tract
- Use of anti-ulcer therapy for any reason
- Simultaneous use of glucocorticoids (steroid drugs like prednisone), particularly in patients with rheumatoid arthritis
- Other medical diseases such as cardiovascular disease
- Patients with severe rheumatoid arthritis
- Large doses of NSAID
- Combinations of NSAIDs

The COX-2 selective drugs were developed to reduce the incidence of these potentially lethal side effects. While most of the media attention has been focused on COX-2 drugs and cardiovascular side effects, a little known fact is that all NSAIDS -regular NSAIDS as well as COX-2 NSAIDS- have the same risk when it comes to heart attack and stroke. This problem extends to the common over the counter NSAIDS such as ibuprofen and naproxyn.

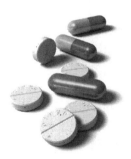

Chapter 36

When are antibiotics used to treat arthritis?

Research has pointed to a possible benefit of using antibiotics for the treatment of some types of arthritis. This article discusses some of the data.

The role of antibiotic therapy for the treatment of arthritis is controversial. However there is at least some evidence for effectiveness in two examples. Minocycline, a member of the tetracycline family, appears to suppress enzymes involved in the inflammatory process. Doxycycline is an antibiotic that also belongs to the tetracycline group and has shown to have positive benefits in osteoarthritis.

Minocycline

In 1949, at the International Congress on Rheumatic Diseases, a possible relationship between mycoplasmas and joint disease was described.

Thomas McPherson Brown, M.D. and his colleagues at the National Institutes of Health reported the following year that rheumatoid arthritis may be caused by an immunologic reaction of antigen and antibody (with mycoplasma as the suspected antigen).

In 1955, Brown reported that mycoplasmas, unlike bacteria and viruses, could live in tissue cell cultures without destroying the tissue cells. In 1964, a high incidence of mycoplasma antibodies in the blood of rheumatoid arthritis patients was found, indicating current or previous infection. Also noted was a four-fold higher incidence of mycoplasma antibodies in females suggesting a correlation with the higher incidence of rheumatoid arthritis in females.

Efforts to demonstrate the effectiveness of tetracycline therapy were initiated and first reported by Dr. Brown shortly thereafter. In 1989, NIH initiated controlled clinical trials of tetracycline therapy for rheumatoid arthritis. The preliminary results of the clinical trials, known now as MIRA or Minocycline in Rheumatoid Arthritis, appeared promising.

The result of the MIRA clinical trial was: "Patients who suffer from mild to moderate RA now have the choice of another therapeutic agent. Not only did the antibiotic significantly reduce symptoms, but side effects were minimal and less severe than observed for most other common rheumatoid treatments."

Despite these findings, many rheumatologists remain skeptical. Other studies have failed to demonstrate clinically significant improvement.

According to the American College of Rheumatology, "Minocycline is prescribed for patients with symptoms of mild rheumatoid arthritis. It is sometimes combined with other medications to treat patients with persistent symptoms of this form of arthritis."

Their formal position is stated in this fact sheet for patients:

...There is evidence minocycline may slow the progression of joint damage in arthritis and prevent disability like other drugs in the class known as DMARDs (disease-modifying anti-rheumatic drugs).

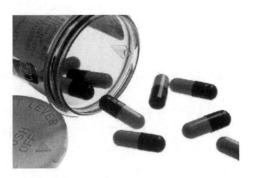

Minocycline is prescribed for patients with symptoms of mild rheumatoid arthritis, sometimes in combination with other medications to treat patients with persistent symptoms of this form of arthritis.

...Minocycline decreases the production of substances causing inflammation, such as prostaglandins and leukotrienes, while increasing production of interleukin-10, a substance that reduces inflammation.

Minocycline usually is given as a 100 milligram (mg) capsule twice a day. It may be taken with food, although it should not be taken with other medications such as antacids or iron tablets.

It may take 2 to 3 months before any improvement in arthritis symptoms is experienced and up to a year before maximum benefits are realized.

The most common side effects from this medicine are gastrointestinal symptoms, dizziness and skin rash. Some women who take minocycline develop vaginal yeast infections. While this can occur with other antibiotics, it seems more prevalent with minocycline and other tetracyclines. It is thought minocycline kills bacteria normally present in the body which protect against yeast infections.

In addition, minocycline may increase sensitivity to sunlight, resulting in more frequent sunburns or the development of rashes following sun exposure. It is recommended therefore, that patients apply sunscreen (SPF 15 or greater) before outdoor activities or avoid prolonged exposure to the sun while taking minocycline.

More rarely, minocycline can affect the kidneys or liver. Doctors may recommend periodic blood tests for long-term users to check liver and kidney function. In equally rare cases, minocycline can induce lupus; fortunately, this potential side effect usually improves after stopping the medication.

Minocyline use during pregnancy can slow the growth of teeth or bones in infants after birth as well as cause discoloration of the newborn's teeth when taken during the last half of pregnancy. Another point... minocycline may decrease the effectiveness of some birth control pills.

Additionally, minocycline is passed into breast milk, so mothers should avoid breast-feeding to prevent delayed development of teeth and bones in their infants. Minocycline can increase a nursing infant's risk of fungal infections or dizziness in the newborn. Because minocycline may cause discoloration of teeth and problems with bone growth in young children, it is recommended that those younger than 8 years old not take this medication. This is not a problem in older children and adults.

Possible interactions with minocycline may occur when taking warfarin (Coumadin), antacids containing calcium, aluminum or magnesium (such as Tums, Rolaids, Maalox, or Mylanta), iron tablets and oral contraceptives (birth control pills).

To highlight one of the potential side effects of minocycline, a small study reported in the June 2006 issue of the Journal of Rheumatology indicated that skin discoloration (hyperpigmentation) appears to be a very common side effect of minocycline use. The study involved 27 patients. Forty-one percent (11 patients) reported developing skin discoloration after using minocycline for approximately one year. Four of the 11 patients stopped using minocycline because of hyperpigmentation (two had skin discoloration on their face and two had skin discoloration on their arms).

The use of minocycline for rheumatoid arthritis is rare nowadays because of the proliferation of newer biologic therapies. Nonetheless, it remains a viable option for the rare individual with extremely mild disease.

Doxycycline

Doxycycline, another tetracycline derivative, has been used to treat osteoarthritis. Study results reported in Arthritis & Rheumatism (July 2005 issue) suggest that treatment with the antibiotic doxycycline may slow the progression of this disease.

Researchers compared the use of doxycycline to placebo, using about 400 obese women with knee arthritis as study participants. Researchers analyzed the impact of doxycycline on the joint space of the affected knee.

The study participants were randomized into two groups, receiving either 100mgs of doxycycline two times a day or placebo for up to two and a half years.

Following 16 months of treatment, results indicated that the average loss of joint space in the affected knee was 40% less among participants taking doxycycline than those who took placebo.

At the end of the two and a half year period, the loss of joint space was 33% less in the group who took doxycyline than in the group who took placebo.

Doxycycline treated patients also reported having marginally less joint pain.

Researchers said that this was the first major study of doxycycline as a potential treatment for osteoarthritis. More studies will be needed to confirm these results.

While the study did not clearly show that oral doxycycline was effective in reducing pain, there was evidence that there was less progression of osteoarthrits (i.e. less cartilage loss) in patients on the antibiotic. The authors felt doxycycline works through anti-inflammatory effect and not due to an anti-bacterial effect.

Based on this study, it is difficult to recommend long term doxycyline for relief of symptoms. On the other hand, it is possible that patients taking the antibiotic may be less likely to require joint replacement in the future due to a decrease in joint damage on radiograph.

Obviously, longer term studies are required. The problem, as it exists today, is that we have no other drugs with significant disease-modifying effects for osteoarthritis.

Chapter 37

How does osteoarthritis develop and what can you do to treat it?

Osteoarthritis is a disease of cartilage. Cartilage is a tough, flexible connective tissue that is found throughout the body. This rubbery tissue which covers the ends of long bones functions mainly as a cushion for joints. It also, because it is covered by a thin layer of lubricating material called "synovial fluid" also acts to allow gliding of joints.

Cartilage does not have a blood or nerve supply... as a result, unlike damaged skin or muscles that can heal, damaged cartilage will not heal quickly and cartilage damage, when it occurs, is not usually painful...

There are three types of cartilage:

- Elastic cartilage is a pliable form of cartilage found in structures such as the outside of the ears, nose, and epiglottis.
- Fibrocartilage is a tough type of cartilage and is very shock resistant. It is found in the discs that form part of the spinal column and also is the type of cartilage that makes up the meniscus (ring of cushion material) located in the knees, hips, and shoulders.
- Hyaline cartilage is a softer type of cartilage that is found most commonly in joints.

Cartilage damage is not painful early on, since no nerve fibers are present. However, as the problem progresses and develops into arthritis, there are symptoms which occur.

Symptoms of articular cartilage damage include:

- decreased range of movement in the affected joint
- joint pain
- stiffness
- swelling

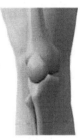

If the damage is particularly severe, a piece of cartilage can break off and become loose. In this case, the loose piece of cartilage may affect the movement of the joint. This can cause a feeling of the joint 'locking' or 'catching'. Sometimes, the joint may also give way.

Articular cartilage damage can occur as a result of trauma- a direct blow to the cartilage. This is why cartilage damage is often a problem for people who play contact sports.

Cartilage can also become damaged gradually, over time. There is an increased risk of developing this type of cartilage damage for heavy individuals, or for people with an anatomic abnormality which causes a structural problem with the joint. This gradual wear and tear is called osteoarthritis.

Interestingly enough, immobility can also damage the cartilage.

The major problem when damage occurs to cartilage is that articular cartilage has a very limited capacity for self repair. A small amount of damage does not repair itself and often gets worse over time.

www.arthritistreatmentcenter.com

The diagnosis of cartilage damage can be suspected by a careful history and physical examination. Confirmation can be obtained by diagnostic studies such as:

- Magnetic resonance imaging (MRI): MRI scans use strong magnetic fields to produce detailed images of the inside of the body. It can often detect cartilage damage.
- Diagnostic ultrasound: This relatively new method of musculoskeletal diagnosis uses sound waves to image cartilage and inflammation.
- Arthroscopy: This is a form of surgery where an arthroscope, a small telescope, is used to look inside the joint.
- X-ray: While this is the traditional method of imaging, the drawback is that osteoarthritis has to be relatively severe before it shows up on x-ray.

There are a number of treatments that can help to relieve the symptoms of damaged articular cartilage. Nonsurgical approaches include:

- Nonsteroidal anti-inflammatory drugs (NSAIDS) help with pain and inflammation. They do have potential side effects that require close monitoring.
- Physical therapy. Various types of treatments such as electrical stimulation, diathermy, and ultrasound can reduce pain. And exercises which strengthen the muscles supporting the joint may help to reduce the pressure on the joint and reduce pain.
- Assistive devices. Canes, walkers, and braces are sometimes useful.
- Lifestyle changes. Weight reduction, regular exercise, and so on can be useful.
- Corticosteroid injections can reduce pain and swelling temporarily but should not be given in the same joint more than 3 times per year.

- Viscosupplements are special lubricants that may dramatically improve pain and mobility when injected into a joint. It is strongly recommended that steroid and viscosupplement injections be given using ultrasound guidance to ensure proper placement of injections.

When non-surgical approaches aren't enough, then surgical treatments may be required.

- Arthroscopic lavage and debridement employs an arthroscope to wash the joint out. The technique cannot repair the damaged cartilage, but it can help to reduce the pain and increase mobility.
- Microfracture surgery: This is a procedure that involves drilling tiny holes (micro fractures) into the bone underneath the damaged cartilage. This exposes the blood vessels inside the bone. Blood cells then begin to stimulate the production of new cartilage. The disadvantage is that the newly formed cartilage is fibrocartilage rather than hyaline cartilage. Fibrocartilage is not as strong as hyaline cartilage. Therefore, it can wear away more quickly than hyaline cartilage.
- Mosaicplasty: This is a technique that involves removing healthy cartilage from the non-weight bearing areas of a joint and using it to replace damaged cartilage.
- Autologous chondrocyte implantation (ACI): This is a technique where a small sample of cartilage cells is taken from the non-weight bearing part of the knee.

The cells are sent to a laboratory where they are stimulated to divide and produce new cells. After a few weeks, the number of cartilage cells will have increased by about 50-100 times from their original number. The new cartilage cells will then be placed under a flap of material that is sewn over the damaged part of the joint.

There are a number of research projects that are currently

investigating additional efficient and effective ways of repairing cartilage.

- Hybrid cartilage is an investigational procedure where human cartilage cells are combined with synthetic fibers to form a patch.
- Stem cells: Another area of research is looking at ways of using special cells, known as mesenchymal stem cells, to generate new cartilage. This latter procedure is promising. Significant improvement in cartilage growth has been demonstrated. Unfortunately, only a few centers worldwide have the knowledge and expertise to perform this procedure properly.

Chapter 38

My doctor wants to give me a cortisone shot... what are the risks?

Cortisone shots are a common procedure given for relief of pain and inflammation. This chapter discusses some of the benefits and dangers.

Natural cortisone is produced by the adrenal glands and is released into the circulation during periods of stress.

Injectable cortisone is produced synthetically and is chemically similar to natural cortisone. Synthetic cortisone is more potent than natural cortisone and is also longer acting.

Cortisone treats inflammation. Injections of cortisone provide a high concentration of drug into a localized area. This "slug" of drug reduces inflammation quickly with few potential side effects. The injections usually work within hours to days and may last several weeks to months.

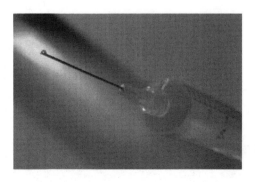

Cortisone injections are used for swollen joints in patients with arthritis and also for bursitis, tendonitis, tennis elbow, trigger finger, and nerve entrapment conditions such as carpal tunnel syndrome.

The shot can be painful but when administered by a skilled practitioner, it usually is well tolerated. Injections for tendonitis can be done with a small gauge needle. Sometimes a larger bore needle is used if the doctor is trying to remove fluid from a swollen joint prior to injecting the cortisone. Often the doctor will "numb the area" either with a freezing spray or with a small injection of a numbing medicine like Lidocaine. Often Lidocaine or Marcaine is injected along with the cortisone to provide temporary relief.

The most common side-effect of a cortisone shot is a "flare." This is a situation where the injected cortisone crystallizes out and causes a short period of intense pain. This usually lasts about a day or two and is best treated by icing the injected area. Another common side effect is lightening discoloration of the skin where the injection is given. This may be a concern in people with darker skin. It is not harmful but patients should be made aware of this.

Other side effects of cortisone injections can be quite serious. A rare but very serious complication is infection, especially if the injection is given into a joint. Prevention is achieved by strict attention to sterile technique with sterilization of the skin using betadine and alcohol. Also, patients with diabetes may have a temporary increase in their blood sugar which they need to be informed about.

True allergic reactions to cortisone are very rare.

Cortisone injections should not be used cavalierly. If one or two injections for a given problem don't work, the injections probably should not be repeated.

No more than three cortisone shots into a given area should be given in a year. Cortisone shots into different areas may be given a bit more often. However, cortisone does have a detrimental effect on tissue. Cortisone has been shown in animal studies to weaken tendons and cause damage to cartilage. Therefore the balance between the relief of symptoms versus the long term effects of cortisone on tissue needs to be balanced.

Chapter 39

Viscosupplements for my knee arthritis - what are they?

In osteoarthritis, the cartilage in the joint gradually wears away. During the course of cartilage degeneration, there is inflammation and resultant stiffness and pain. Osteoarthritis may be caused by, or aggravated, by excess stress on the joint from deformity, repeated trauma, or excess weight. It most often affects middle aged and older people.

A younger person who develops osteoarthritis may have an inherited form of the disease or may have experienced problems as a result of injury.

In rheumatoid arthritis, the joint becomes inflamed and cartilage may be destroyed as well. Arthritis not only affects joints, it can also affect supporting structures such as:

- muscles
- tendons
- ligaments

Rheumatoid arthritis often affects people at an earlier age than osteoarthritis.

Regardless of the type of arthritis causing knee symptoms, the end result is often the same. A person who has arthritis in the knee may experience pain, swelling, and a decrease in knee motion. A common symptom is morning stiffness that gets better as the person moves around. Sometimes the joint locks or clicks when the knee is bent and straightened, but these signs may occur in other knee disorders as well.

The doctor may confirm the diagnosis by performing a physical examination and examining magnetic resonance (MR) scans, which reveal the inner architecture of the knee.

Most often arthritis in the knee is treated initially with pain-reducing medicines, such as analgesics and anti-inflammatory medicines.

Exercise is essential to restore joint movement and strengthen the knee. Losing excess weight can also help people with osteoarthritis.

Glucocorticoid injections are helpful when there is evidence of inflammation.

The normal knee joint produces synovial fluid, a thick slippery substance that nourishes cartilage and allows smooth gliding of the cartilage surfaces. With arthritis, the amount of synovial fluid made by the joint is reduced.

In instances when other therapies do not provide the desired relief, viscosupplements are sometimes used. These are gel-like substances (hyaluronates) that mimic the properties of naturally occurring joint fluid.

These hyaluronates actually supplement the viscous properties of synovial fluid. Injection of hyaluronates is done using either fluoroscopic or ultrasound needle guidance.

Currently, hyaluronate injections are approved for the treatment of osteoarthritis of the knee in those who have failed to respond to more conservative therapy. The number of injections performed varies with the type of viscosupplement used. Usually five injections are required for the best response.

Currently, there are five FDA approved hyaluronates:

- Hyalgan

- Synvisc
- Euflexa
- Supartz
- Orthovisc

Sometimes, a physician will perform an arthroscopy before providing viscosupplement. Also, a special type of brace to help unload the narrowed part of the knee may be used to help the viscosupplement work better.

Use for other joints is being studied. Studies have shown effectiveness for the shoulder, hip, and ankle. We published a study a few years ago showing these viscosupplements are effective for osteoarthritis affecting the base of the thumb.

Chapter 40

What you need to know about food and drug interactions if you have arthritis

Medicines can treat and often cure many medical problems. However they must be taken properly to ensure they are safe and effective. Many medicines have powerful ingredients that interact with the human body in different ways. This article discusses some important information for arthritis sufferers.

Medications often interact with food. Both food, the timing of food intake, as well as lifestyle can impact a drug's ability to work in the body. Certain foods, beverages, alcohol, caffeine, and even cigarettes can interact with medicines. This may make them less effective or may cause dangerous side effects.

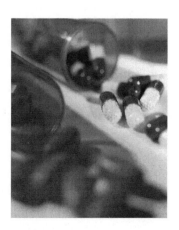

When you take medicine, be sure to follow the doctor's and pharmacist's instructions carefully to obtain the maximum benefit with the least risk. Factors that influence a drug's effects on the body include interaction with food, alcohol, and caffeine as well as other factors such as dose, age, weight, gender, and overall health.

So let's talk about the major category of medicines used to treat arthritis conditions.

Analgesic medicines treat pain. An example is acetaminophen. For rapid relief, take this medicine on an empty stomach because food may allow the body to absorb acetaminophen. Avoid or limit the use of alcohol because the combination of alcohol with acetaminophen can cause damage to the liver.

Nonsteroidal anti-inflammatory drugs (NSAIDs) reduce pain and inflammation. However, because these medicines potentially can irritate the stomach, it is best to take them with food or milk.

Avoid or limit the use of alcohol because chronic alcohol intake can increase the risk of stomach bleeding or liver damage.

Corticosteroids are used to reduce inflammation. These drugs should be taken with food or milk to reduce stomach upset. Corticosteroids taken along with NSAIDS are a particularly harmful combination for the stomach.

Narcotic analgesics provide relief from moderate to severe pain. Some of these drugs are also used in combination with acetaminophen, aspirin, or in cough syrups. Use these medicines with caution because they may become habit forming or cause serious side effects such as liver damage, dizziness, or drowsiness. Avoid alcohol because it increases the sedative effects of these medicines.

Non-narcotic analgesics such as tramadol should also be taken with food since stomach upset is not uncommon.

www.arthritistreatmentcenter.com

Methotrexate, azathioprine (Imuran), hydroxychloroquine (Plaquenil), and sulfasalazine (Azulfidine) are disease-modifying anti-rheumatic drugs (DMARDs). These drugs slow down the progression of arthritis. These drugs may be taken with food but also may cause nausea. Split-dosing these medicines, meaning taking half the dose in the morning and the other half in the evening, may help alleviate the nausea.

However, if you feel really sick, you should contact your physician since severe nausea may be an indication of an allergic reaction.

Some drugs, such as cyclosporine, should not be taken with grapefruit juice or taken when a patient is eating grapefruit because there may be problems with drug metabolism and cyclosporine may not be able to be excreted in a timely fashion.

Alcohol should be strictly limited if you take these drugs particularly if you are taking methotrexate because of the danger of toxicity to the liver.

In patients with co-morbid conditions (i.e. other medical conditions), the combination of medicines required for different conditions can also lead to problems with drug-drug interaction. It is important that patients with arthritis who are taking multiple medicines coordinate their medicines with their various physicians.

Chapter 41

For rheumatoid arthritis sufferers... Some info about methotrexate

Rheumatoid arthritis is the most common inflammatory form of arthritis. It affects more than two million Americans. Because it is a systemic disease capable of damaging internal organs, it must be, and usually is, treated very aggressively.

The most widely prescribed disease-modifying anti-rheumatic drug (DMARD) for rheumatoid arthritis is methotrexate.

Methotrexate has been in use since the early 1980's and is the "gold standard" by which rheumatologists judge all other DMARDs. It is also the drug upon which other medicines such as biologic response modifiers (BRMs) are added.

Methotrexate interferes with folic acid metabolism by blocking a specific enzyme called dihydrofolate reductase. Dihydrofolate reductase is required for the growth of actively dividing cells. Since inflammation is perpetuated by rapidly growing cells, methotrexate is felt to exert its effects by blocking the multiplication or proliferation of these cells.

As a result of its actions, methotrexate reduces the swelling and pain associated with rheumatoid arthritis and also decreases the risk of long term disability. It takes roughly 4 to 12 weeks to see the maximum effects of methotrexate. During this short period of time, the dose of methotrexate is started low and gradually increased.

The drug can be administered in several ways. Patients who have extremely active disease can be treated intravenously to help with induction of remission. Patients can then be treated with oral tablets. The tablets come in a dose of 2.5mg per tablet. Methotrexate is taken as a single dose of medicine once a week. That means if a patient is taking the drug either intravenously or in tablet form, they take all their medicine at one time once a week. Some patients who have difficulty taking oral tablets because of nausea may be able to take their methotrexate as a subcutaneous injection.

The dose of methotrexate varies from as low as 5mg per week to as high as 25mg per week. Doses higher than 25mg tend to be poorly tolerated.

Potential side effects include mouth sores, gastrointestinal problems such as nausea, vomiting, and diarrhea, shortness of breath, cough, liver function abnormalities, hair loss, sun sensitivity, and decrease in white blood cell count or platelet count. Rarely, cirrhosis of the liver can occur. Older people who have dietary deficiencies are at particular risk for methotrexate side effects.

Patients should have laboratory testing of blood counts and liver function tests once a month.

Patients are usually given supplemental folic acid in a dose of 1-2mg per day to counteract some of the side effects of methotrexate.

www.arthritistreatmentcenter.com

Methotrexate is terribly teratogenic (capable of causing birth defects). Therefore, women, as well as men, who are contemplating having children, need to hold their methotrexate for at least three months prior to attempting conception.

Since methotrexate is capable of damaging the liver, patients should be counseled about limiting or eliminating alcohol ingestion.

Furthermore, methotrexate can interact with a number of other medicines including antibiotics such as sulfa drugs as well as nonsteroidal anti-inflammatory drugs.

Methotrexate is often used in combination with biologic drugs such as Enbrel, Humira, and Remicade.

Chapter 43

I'm confused about all the medicines used to treat rheumatoid arthritis... Can you explain them to me?

Part 1: The anti-inflammatory and glucorticoid group

Rheumatoid arthritis (RA) is a chronic, potentially destructive, systemic, autoimmune form of arthritis. It affects roughly two million Americans and has been the subject of intense research, particularly in recent years.

The goal of treatment is to induce remission. This chapter is on anti-inflammatory drugs and glucocorticoid medicines used to treat RA.

The first group of medicines that are often employed are anti-inflammatory drugs. Salicylates (aspirin), nonsteroidal anti-inflammatory drugs (NSAIDs), or selective cyclooxygenase COX-2 inhibitors (eg., Celebrex) may reduce joint pain and swelling and improve joint function. These agents have analgesic and anti-inflammatory properties but do not alter the course of the disease or prevent joint destruction. As a result, they should not be used as the only treatment for RA.

Patients with RA are nearly twice as likely as patients with other forms of arthritis, such as osteoarthritis, to have a serious complication from NSAID treatment. Serious gastrointestinal side effects, such as bleeding, ulcers, and perforation of the stomach, small intestine, or large intestine can occur at any time, with or without warning symptoms, in patients treated with NSAIDs (including COX-2 inhibitors, particularly if patients are taking concurrent aspirin).

Risk factors for the NSAID-associated ulcers affecting the stomach or duodenum (the first part of the small intestine) include age older than 75 years, history of ulcer, associated use of steroids or blood thinners, higher dosage of NSAIDs, use of multiple NSAIDs, and a serious underlying disease.

In 2005, the American College of Rheumatology (ACR) added to their 2002 RA treatment guidelines the warning that some placebo-controlled trials showed an increased risk for cardiovascular events, including non-fatal heart attacks and strokes, with COX-2 selective NSAIDs, particularly when used at higher doses.

Obviously, physicians and patients need to weigh the potential risks and benefits of treatment with these medications.

Glucocorticoids ("steroids") are often used early in the treatment of active RA. They have potent anti-inflammatory effects and are effective in reducing symptoms quickly.

Glucocorticoids are often started at the same time as other medicines, the disease-modifying anti-rheumatic drugs (DMARDs), are started. This is because steroids act quickly while DMARDs act much more slowly.

In this instance, glucocorticoids are used as a "bridge" to help a patient with their symptoms quickly while waiting for DMARDs to kick in.

Frequently, disabling recurrence of joint inflammation returns when glucocorticoids are discontinued, even in patients who are receiving DMARDs. Therefore, many patients with RA are dependent on glucocorticoids and continue them long term. That's the bad news.

The good news is that some recent evidence suggests that low-dose glucocorticoids slow the rate of joint damage and appear to have disease-modifying potential. Joint damage may increase on discontinuation of glucocorticoids. The benefits of low-dose systemic glucocorticoids should always be weighed against their adverse effects. The adverse effects of long-term oral glucocorticoids even at low doses include osteoporosis, hypertension, weight gain, fluid retention, elevated blood sugar, cataracts, and thin skin, as well as the potential for premature hardening of the arteries. These potential side effects should be considered and discussed in detail with the patient before glucocorticoid therapy is begun.

For long term disease control, the glucocorticoid dosage should be kept to a minimum. For most patients with RA, this means less than 7.5-10mg of prednisone per day.

RA is associated with an increased risk for osteoporosis independent of glucocorticoid therapy. Some patients may require injections of glucocorticoids into joints to help with painful flares. Joint infection needs to be ruled out before local glucocorticoid injections are given. As a rule, the same joint should not be injected more than once within three months.

These drugs, while important, must be used in combination with DMARDs and biologic therapies. These drugs will be discussed in parts 2 and 3 of this series.

Chapter 44

I'm confused about all the medicines used to treat rheumatoid arthritis... Can you explain them to me?

Part 2: The disease-modifying anti-rheumatic drug (DMARD) group

Rheumatoid arthritis (RA) is a chronic, potentially destructive, systemic, autoimmune form of arthritis. It affects roughly two million Americans and has been the subject of intense research, particularly in recent years.

The goal of treatment is to induce remission.

In a previous chapter, I discussed the use of nonsteroidal anti-inflammatory drugs (NSAIDS) and glucocorticoids in rheumatoid arthritis (RA). In this chapter I will discuss disease-modifying anti-rheumatic drugs (DMARDs).

Although nonsteroidal anti-inflammatory drugs (NSAIDs) and glucocorticoids ("steroids") may alleviate symptoms, joint damage can progress in patients with active rheumatoid arthritis (RA). Disease-modifying anti-rheumatic drugs (DMARDs) can reduce or prevent joint damage, preserve joint integrity and function, and maintain the economic productivity of the patient with RA.

DMARD therapy should be considered in all patients with active RA. DMARD therapy should be started immediately -certainly within three months of diagnosis- in any patient who has persistent joint pain, significant morning stiffness or fatigue, active joint inflammation, persistent elevation of the ESR (sed rate) or CRP level (these latter two are blood tests that measure inflammation), or x-ray joint damage.

For any untreated patient with persistent joint inflammation and joint damage, DMARD treatment should be started to prevent or slow further damage. Unfortunately, all DMARDs including methotrexate (MTX), sulfasalazine (SSZ), hydroxychloroquine (HCQ), leflunomide, azathioprine, cyclophosphamide, and cyclosporine require several weeks to months before improvement begins to occur.

Most rheumatologists select MTX as their initial DMARD, particularly for patients where the RA is active. Because of its efficacy, relatively low toxicity, and low cost, MTX has become the standard by which all DMARDs are compared.

Controlled clinical trials have established the efficacy of MTX in RA, particularly in patients with severe disease. MTX slows the progression of x-ray damage, and more than 50% of patients who take MTX continue the drug beyond three years. Mouth sores, nausea, diarrhea, fatigue, and hair loss caused by MTX can be reduced by treating the patient with folic acid supplementation.

Relative contraindications for MTX therapy are pregnancy (MTX is a potent teratogen, meaning it causes severe birth defects), pre-existing liver disease (especially infectious hepatitis), kidney function impairment, significant lung disease, and alcohol abuse.

A liver biopsy should be considered in patients who develop abnormal findings on blood liver function tests that persist during treatment or after discontinuation of MTX where no other cause for the abnormalities are found.

MTX can be used either by itself (monotherapy) or in combination with another DMARD.

In some patients, as described above, MTX is contraindicated. Not all people respond to MTX and some people are unable to tolerate it.

In that case, other DMARDs can be used.

Hydroxychloroquine (Plaquenil) is a mild DMARD that may decrease the pain and swelling of arthritis as well as reduce the risk for long-term disability. It can be used early in the course of RA and is often used in combination with other DMARDs. Taking a high dose for prolonged periods has been associated with damage to the retina, and an eye examination is recommended for most patients every 6 to 12 months.

Sulfasalazine (SSZ) is a sulfa-based DMARD. It acts more quickly than hydroxychloroquine, sometimes as early as four weeks. SSZ can slow x-ray progression of RA and is usually well tolerated. Most adverse effects (nausea and stomach discomfort) occur in the first few months of therapy. Starting low and gradually increasing the dosage lessens the incidence of these adverse effects. Low white blood cell counts can occur and may be serious. Periodic laboratory monitoring is necessary. Clinical response should be apparent within three months.

Leflunomide (Arava) has a slightly different mechanism of action than MTX and is taken in pill form once a day. It can be used alone or with MTX, although the risk for adverse effects (including liver problems) is greater with this combination. The reduction in disease activity and in the rate of x-ray progression by leflunomide alone is equal to that of MTX. As with MTX, liver tests must be monitored closely. Five percent of patients receiving leflunomide and up to 60% of patients receiving MTX plus leflunomide have elevated liver enzyme levels.

Leflunomide is a potent teratogen - it causes severe birth defects. If a patient is planning pregnancy, the drug should be stopped and cholestyramine elimination performed (cholestyramine 8gm three times daily by mouth for 11 days).

Adherence to the package insert on ridding leflunomide from the system is mandatory before pregnancy is considered.

Other DMARDs occasionally used in RA include azathioprine (Imuran), cyclosporine (Sandimmune), and gold therapy (Solganol, Myochrisine). Azathioprine and cyclosporine are immunosuppressant drugs taken in pill form. The usual dose for azathioprine is once daily, whereas cyclosporine is generally started at twice daily. Intramuscular gold injection is typically initiated as a low test dose followed by a higher weekly dose over 5-6 months.

While many rheumatologists select hydroxychloroquine or sulfasalazine first, MTX is usually preferred.

After five years, only 60% of patients remain on MTX, the best-tolerated traditional DMARD. Joint damage by x-ray is found in 30% of patients after one year of therapy with traditional DMARDs and in 70% of patients after two years of therapy. Joint damage by x-ray is closely correlated with subsequent disability. In addition, significant numbers of patients on DMARD therapy may still have progressive x-ray damage and disability.

Numerous studies have established the importance of aggressive DMARDs as single-drugs and as combination agent treatments. The existence of a window of opportunity is now a well accepted concept in RA therapeutics. This window consists of the first 3-6 months of disease and is the best time to initiate therapy to prevent x-ray damage and subsequent disability. A number of controlled studies have recommended the use of early aggressive DMARD therapy either alone or in combination.

Chapter 44

I'm confused about all the medicines used to treat rheumatoid arthritis... Can you explain them to me?

Part 3: The biologics

Rheumatoid arthritis (RA) is a chronic, potentially destructive, systemic, autoimmune form of arthritis. It affects roughly two million Americans and has been the subject of intense research, particularly in recent years.

The goal of treatment is to induce remission.

In previous chapters, I discussed nonsteroidal anti-inflammatory drugs (NSAIDs) and disease-modifying anti-rheumatic drugs (DMARDs) and their role in rheumatoid arthritis. This chapter will talk about the biologic group.

Of all the advances in treatment for rheumatoid arthritis (RA), none has had a greater impact than the biologics.

Biologics are drugs that are made from living sources (hence the term "biologic") such as humans, animals, or microorganisms, and are grown in specially engineered cells. They differ from conventional medicines which are developed through chemical reactions in the laboratory.

The first biologics were vaccines. Probably the earliest credible account of a vaccine was the one produced in the laboratory by Louis Pasteur in 1879.

A few short years later Banting and Best were able to isolate insulin, another biologic used to treat diabetes.

Blood and blood products such as plasma, white cells, and platelets are also considered biologic treatments.

The biologics that have most recently been created have been derived through sophisticated biotechnological research techniques using genetic material, DNA, and cell fusion techniques.

The biologics of today are called "large molecule" drugs. They are not only larger in molecule size and number but are also more complex in general compared with conventional drugs ("small molecule" drugs). Small molecule drugs consist of drugs that contain between 20 to 100 atoms. An example would be aspirin, which has 21 atoms. These drugs can be taken orally.

Because of their large size, biologics typically are injected subcutaneously or intramuscularly or are infused intravenously.

Biologic drugs have revolutionized the treatment of diseases such as rheumatoid arthritis, psoriatic arthritis, ankylosing spondylitis, and systemic lupus erythematosus.

Most of the biologic drugs used for arthritis treatment were first applied in RA and then further research lead to approval for other rheumatic diseases.

Examples of biologic drugs used to treat arthritis include anti-TNF drugs such as etanercept (Enbrel), adalimumab (Humira), infliximab (Remicade), golimumab (Simponi), and certolizumab (Cimzia); anti-IL-1 drugs like anakinra (Kineret); IL-6 blockers like tocilizumab

(Actemra); anti B-cell therapies like rituximab (Rituxan); and T-cell co-stimulatory blockers like abatacept (Orencia).

Using both clinical as well as laboratory measurements, physicians have been able to demonstrate remarkable disease response to these new agents. Prior to the use of biologic drugs, it was unusual for rheumatologists to talk about remission. Nowadays, it is usually possible to achieve remission.

Biologic drugs do have potential side effects that limit their effectiveness. The first is increased incidence of infections in patients receiving biologics. The second is drug toxicity. The last is the development of antibodies to the biologic.

Because there are many patients who fail biologics because of allergic reactions, primary failure (don't respond at all), secondary failure (respond initially, but then fail), and drug toxicity, further research is being conducted to develop drugs with other mechanisms of action.

Multiple randomized, double-blind, placebo-controlled trials have demonstrated the efficacy of the anti-TNF (tumor necrosis factor) agents in improving clinical symptoms and signs in patients with RA.

Patients with early RA, as well as those with active RA in whom previous DMARD therapy has failed, show improvement with TNF inhibitors. These agents have been shown to be beneficial when used in combination with methotrexate (MTX) in patients with ongoing active RA despite adequate doses of MTX alone. TNF-inhibitors block the effects of tumor necrosis factor which plays a major role in the perpetuation of inflammation and joint damage in RA.

Many patients improve rapidly even during the first two weeks. Also, there is less x-ray progression with these agents after one year than in patients treated with MTX alone.

In one study, the early treatment of RA with adalimumab plus methotrexate versus adalimumab alone or MTX alone demonstrated the effectiveness of aggressive MTX combined with an anti-TNF medicine versus either single drug alone with respect to clinical, functional, and x-ray outcomes.

Several studies have also demonstrated the effectiveness of these drugs in later disease as well. The TNF inhibitors adalimumab and etanercept are given subcutaneously every 1-2 weeks. The third drug, infliximab, requires intravenous infusions initially, then at two weeks, six weeks, and then every eight weeks. In addition, it needs to be given with weekly MTX to lower the incidence of antibodies produced against infliximab. Antibody production occurs because infliximab has mouse proteins that the body recognizes as foreign. The normal immune response is then to mount a gradual antibody response to the drug.

Anakinra (Kineret) is a subcutaneously administered biologic drug that blocks a protein called interleukin (IL)-1. It needs to be given daily as a subcutaneous injection. It appears to work less well than the anti-TNF drugs. It should not be given along with a TNF inhibitor because of an unacceptably high rate of infection with such a combination.

Tocilizumab (Actemra) is a drug that blocks interleukin 6, a cytokine that promotes inflammation. Actemra was approved by the FDA in early 2010 and is effective for use in patients with rheumatoid arthritis who have failed TNF inhibitors. I generally use it in combination with methotrexate. It has a side effect profile similar to that of other biologic therapies. Elevations in liver enzymes and blood lipids have been seen. Rare instances of bowel perforation have been reported. The drug is administered intravenously every four weeks.

Abatacept (Orencia) is a T-cell costimulation modulator. It must be given by infusion and is not indicated for same time use with anti-TNF drugs nor with anakinra. Immunizations should be avoided during use and for three months after having stopped this drug. Also, patients with chronic obstructive pulmonary disease experience a higher rate of complications than do those on placebo.

Rituximab (Rituxan) acts through depletion of CD20+ B cells. It is useful for patients who have failed anti-TNF therapy and DMARD therapy. However, side effects include generalized mouth sores and skin rash as well as fatal infusion reactions. The infusion reaction has been seen mostly in patients who have received rituximab for treatment of non-Hodgkins lymphoma. It is much less common in patients with RA. About 80% of infusion reactions occur with the first infusion.

Several trials have shown the value of switching to a different anti-TNF agent or to abatacept or rituximab after initial anti-TNF failure.

Newer treatments including interleukin-6 inhibitors, and oral kinase inhibitors also show promise.

General precautions include the avoidance of live vaccines in any patient receiving a biologic treatment. Combinations of biologics, while intellectually appealing, have not been shown to be any more effective and have actually been shown to cause a higher rate of side effects.

Chapter 45

My doctor wants to start me on Enbrel... What are the risks?

Enbrel (etanercept) is a biologic drug. Biologic drugs are protein-based medications that have been synthesized in a lab to perform a biologic function. Enbrel is a biologic that blocks the effects of tumor necrosis factor-alpha. Tumor necrosis factor (TNF) is a protein messenger produced by immune cells. It promotes and perpetuates inflammation in rheumatoid arthritis (RA).

In addition to Enbrel, there are four other inhibitors of TNF available. They are Remicade (infliximab), Humira (adalimumab), Simponi (golimumab), and Cimzia (certolizumab). All five drugs neutralize and eliminate excess amounts of TNF from the circulation and from areas of inflammation. These cytokine inhibitors have proven effective when other medicines such as disease-modifying anti-rheumatic drugs (DMARDS) like methotrexate have failed to control symptoms or halt joint damage.

They are effective in improving symptomatic and x-ray outcomes and have been found safe, even when administered early in the disease process. However, as these drugs are used more extensively, there are growing concerns about the safety of biologic therapies.

Infection.

Since TNF also helps maintain normal immune function, blocking this cytokine may predispose a patient to infection, malignancy, or other auto-immune states. To date, the most frequently reported adverse events (AEs) are related to the drug's administration -- mild rash, local pain or swelling at administration sites, and hypersensitivity reactions.

Data from the clinical trials for all 3 currently available TNF inhibitors did not show an overall increase in TNF inhibitor-related serious infection rates compared to the placebo control group.

However, several studies have examined drug safety in patients with other underlying diseases and conditions (elderly age, diabetes, chronic lung and kidney disease, chronic osteomyelitis, etc.). This group mirrors the type of patient seen in real life clinical practice.

Results from some of these studies showed an increased risk for infection. In addition, rheumatoid arthritis itself may increase the risk of infection, therefore, confounding the issue.

Data since FDA approval has also shown higher incidences of other types of unusual infections such as tuberculosis, atypical mycobacteria, histoplasmosis, aspergillosis, etc.

These infections appear to be more aggressive and tend to occur in areas of the body outside of the lung. Of greater concern is that infection risk is significantly greater when biologics are given in combination. For instance, the incidence of serious infections was considerably increased when TNF blockers were given along with with Kineret (anakinra) or Orencia (abatacept), and the combination of biologics failed to demonstrate any added benefit over a single drug given alone. Therefore, combination biologic therapy should not be used in patients with RA.

Malignancy.

In addition to infection, there have been concerns that the TNF inhibitor may lead to a greater risk for malignancy, particularly lymphoma, because TNF is an important component of the immune system. Several studies have revealed that patients with RA have an activity-related increased rate of non-Hodgkin's lymphoma compared to that in the normal population. In other words, the worse the RA, the higher the likelihood of developing lymphoma.

www.arthritistreatmentcenter.com

In some studies there has been reported a slightly higher incidence of lymphoma in patients receiving anti-TNF drugs versus patients with RA who don't. However, there may be a selection bias. Patients at highest risk for lymphoma (e.g. those with higher disease activity) are more likely to receive anti-TNF therapy.

Liver and blood problems.

Large clinical studies have also demonstrated evidence of blood count abnormalities and liver enzyme elevations. These abnormalities are difficult to interpret because other factors such as concurrent diseases and concomitant use of medications (e.g. nonsteroidal anti-inflammatory drugs, methotrexate, and leflunomide) may also cause these effects.

Given the potential for blood and liver toxicity, regular laboratory monitoring should be considered for patients receiving TNF inhibitors. More reports are emerging regarding rapidly progressive liver failure in patients with chronic hepatitis B virus infection.

Reactivation of the hepatitis B virus following immunosuppression, leading to fatal hepatitis, has occurred in transplant and cancer patients. Pre-treatment blood testing for chronic viral hepatitis (HBV and hepatitis C virus) is recommended. Prophylaxis with lamivudine or other effective anti-viral drugs should be considered in patients who are hepatitis B surface antigen (HBsAg)-positive and who will be placed on TNF inhibitor therapy.

Congestive heart failure.

Use of TNF inhibitors in patients with moderate to severe congestive heart failure has been discouraged because of the potential for worsening of heart function. TNF may play a role in the progression of heart failure.

Caution should be taken when using TNF inhibitors in patients with unstable cardiac dysfunction.

Other risks.

Demyelinating diseases, lupus-like syndromes, and abnormal antibody production have been reported in association with these drugs. The cases are rare, and the impact of these drugs in patients with other underlying autoimmune conditions such as multiple sclerosis, systemic lupus erythematosus is still unclear.

So… while anti-TNF drugs have revolutionized our ability to treat RA and have allowed us to put significant numbers of patients with RA into remission, they should be used by experienced rheumatologists. Patient education is critical as well.

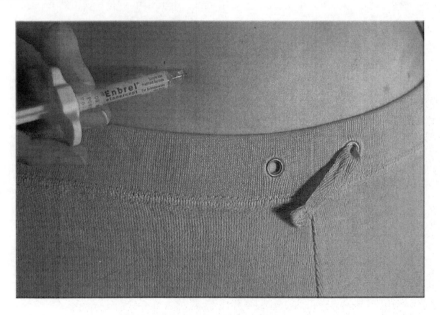

Chapter 46

Do anti-TNF drugs help rheumatoid arthritis patients live longer?

One of the biggest questions when it comes to anti-tumor necrosis therapy (anti-TNF) is... what is the overall risk/benefit ratio? There is no question that this group of drugs induces positive clinical responses in most patients. However, there remains concern about toxicity, including potential problems such as infection and malignancy.

One method of assessing the risk/benefit ratio could be the measurement of overall mortality or rate of death. On the one hand, by effectively controlling systemic inflammation, treatment with TNF blockers could potentially improve mortality. It has been established that patients with the most severe RA have increased mortality. On the other hand, if serious adverse effects due to these drugs were common, this could have a negative effect on overall mortality.

So far, most studies appear to show that treatment with TNF blockers has a beneficial effect on mortality.

Data from one study analyzed 22,545 RA patients from across the United States, over 85,691 patient-years of follow-up (Michaud K, Wolfe F. Reduced mortality among RA patients treated with anti-TNF therapy and methotrexate. Program and abstracts of the American College of Rheumatology 2005 Annual Scientific Meeting; November 13-17, 2005; San Diego, California. Abstract 296).

The 1,713 deaths in this population group were analyzed to determine causes and other factors that might have contributed to death.

Compared with patients not receiving TNF blockers or methotrexate (MTX), the use of TNF blockers, the use of MTX, and the use of TNF blockers plus MTX were all associated with statistically significantly lower risks for death.

Also, a large Swedish study examined 1,534 patients, 949 of whom were on TNF blockers. This population group was scrutinized for factors associated with mortality. Overall, patients on TNF blockers had a slightly lower mortality rate that was not statistically significant compared with those not on TNF blockers. However, when adjusted for disease severity, using the Health Assessment Questionnaire score, TNF blocker treated patients had a significantly lower mortality (Jacobsson LTH, Turesson C, Nilsson L, et al. Treatment with TNF-blockers is associated with reduced premature mortality in patients with rheumatoid arthritis. Program and abstracts of EULAR 2006: 7th Annual European Congress of Rheumatology; June 21-24, 2006; Amsterdam, The Netherlands. Abstract).

This encouraging data should not induce a cavalier response by rheumatologists about this group of medicines. Anti-TNF drugs are a wonderful development; however, close observation of patients on these drugs is mandatory.

Chapter 47

What are the treatment options for rheumatoid arthritis if anti-TNF drugs don't work?

Rheumatoid arthritis (RA) is a chronic, progressive, autoimmune disease that causes both destructive joint changes as well as damage to internal organs.

The advent of drugs that block tumor necrosis factor such as Enbrel, Humira, Remicade, and now Simponi and Cimzia, has revolutionized our approach to the disease. However, what happens if these drugs don't work?

A review by M Asif A Siddiqui in the May 15, 2007 issue of Current Opinion in Rheumatology had some useful information. I will summarize the implications in this chapter.

In long-standing RA, both rituximab (Rituxan), a drug that depletes B lymphocytes, as well as abatacept (Orencia), a drug that inhibits T-cell functioning, in combination with methotrexate provide effective alternative options to anti-TNF drugs in the treatment of signs and symptoms in patients with methotrexate-resistant disease.

Another new drug, tocilizumab (Actemra), a drug that blocks interleukin-6, also appears to be effective in these patients.

Rituximab and abatacept, in combination with methotrexate, were also effective when therapy with anti-TNF agents had not produced an adequate response.

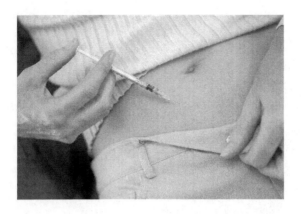

In addition, abatacept taken in combination with methotrexate has been shown to slow the x-ray progression of methotrexate-resistant disease. Rituximab plus methotrexate may also improve x-ray progression of long-standing RA that does not respond adequately to anti-TNF therapy.

However, there is no advantage in adding abatacept to ongoing anti-TNF therapy. In fact, there is an increase in infectious complications with the combination. Other combinations of biologics involving different mechanisms of action have not been explored.

In early, aggressive RA, only tocilizumab monotherapy (single drug) has been evaluated, and has shown to be effective in reducing x-ray progression of RA in one study, but this needs to be confirmed in well designed trials.

The newer biologics appear to be well tolerated, with an acceptable tolerability profile. More studies with longer follow-up times are needed.

Based on the evidence, the safe and effective dosages of abatacept, rituximab, and tocilizumab appear to be 10mg/kg, 500 and 1000mg, and 8mg/kg, respectively. Rituximab may have an advantage in terms of its schedule, since a single course consisting of two infusions two weeks apart produces a beneficial effect that can be sustained for up to one year, and sometimes longer. However, the safety of repeat courses of rituximab needs to be assessed.

Oral drugs directed against protein kinases also look promising. The newer biologics are a useful and very welcome addition to the therapeutic arsenal employed against RA.

Chapter 48

My doctor has told me I need a joint replacement. What questions do I need to ask?

More than 300,000 hip and knee replacements are performed in the United States each year. Less commonly, other joints such as the shoulder, elbow, and fingers are replaced.

These surgical procedures replace the diseased joint surfaces with plastic, metal or ceramic surfaces. The technical term for this type of procedure is a "total joint arthroplasty."

Before undergoing any surgical procedure, a patient should be certain that all non-surgical options have been tried.

What these options may be depends upon the type of arthritis being treated.

For rheumatoid arthritis, a patient should have been treated with non-steroidal anti-inflammatory drugs, low dose corticosteroids, methotrexate, and biologic agents along with physical therapy.

For patients with osteoarthritis the usual non-surgical treatments are analgesic (pain-killing) drugs, nonsteroidal-anti-inflammatory drugs and physical therapy.

With both types of arthritis, injecting the damaged joint with medications -glucocorticoids or viscosupplements (lubricating medications)- is often very helpful.

www.arthritistreatmentcenter.com

Arthroscopic treatment- (going into the joint using a small telescope-with removal of damaged and diseased tissue) can sometimes afford relief.

More recently, stem cell procedures designed to regrow cartilage have shown much promise.

Once you and your doctor determine surgery is the appropriate treatment, you should fully understand all the components of the operation and remember that every surgical procedure entails risk. Among the more serious risks are allergic reactions to anesthesia, excessive bleeding, infection, and blood clots. There is also a chance the replacement surgery won't relieve the pain. The chances for complications increase if you have other complicated medical problems.

You should also ask about the surgeon's experience. A joint replacement surgeon should specialize in joint replacements and do them all the time. You want a pro, not a person who does these every so often. Ask who will be doing the surgery. If you are at a teaching hospital, you may have a resident doing it. This is no knock against the resident but you should make sure the attending surgeon is there too.

If you have two knees that need to be replaced, ask if both can be done at the same time.

Most important, patients should ask what will be expected of them after surgery. What will the rehabilitation entail? How long is the hospital stay? What are my needs when I go home? Most centers that specialize in joint replacement surgery will have a comprehensive program that will address these needs.

Chapter 49

I have arthritis... What are my options for joint replacement?

The two most common joints that are replaced for arthritis related problems are the hip and the knee.

Two major types of joint replacements are available.

The first type is the cemented joint. In this procedure, the artificial joint is glued to the natural bone.

The other type is the uncemented. Here, the replacement joint is covered with a porous textured material and natural bone then grows and attaches to the joint replacement.

Roughly, 90 percent of artificial joints last 10 to 15 years after which a second joint replacement, otherwise known as a "revision" is then required.

Cemented joints are generally offered to patients with osteoporosis, because the cement holds the artificial joint in place more firmly. These types of replacements are more difficult to revise than uncemented ones because the cement needs to be removed. Cemented artificial joints are generally used for frailer and older individuals who are likely to have less bone mass and are also less likely to require a revision procedure. The main problem with cemented joints is that some of them loosen over time and need revision.

Uncemented artificial joints are a better choice for younger, healthier, more active people. These individuals are more likely to require a revision procedure down the road. They also have denser bones which keep the artificial joint anchored more firmly. Approximately 30 per cent of patients who receive an uncemented joint for hip arthritis develop thigh pain. This problem may last for as long as two to three years after surgery. Uncemented hip replacements take longer to heal and patients require a longer period of time before they can begin to bear weight. Too much stress on the uncemented joint too early leads to loosening.

Full recovery takes about 6 months for both procedures.

Serious complications occur in about 5 percent of people receiving joint replacements. The most frequent is thrombophlebitis (blood clots in the legs). The danger is that these blood clots can travel to the lungs. This is called a pulmonary embolism and is potentially life-threatening. Attempts to prevent this complication have been successful in many instances. These include the use of aspirin, heparin or other blood thinners, and leg compression devices. These leg compression units inflate and deflate so that the leg is constantly massaged.

Another potentially serious complication is infection. This side effect requires both removal of the artificial joint as well as treatment with intravenous antibiotics. The treatment requires several weeks of hospitalization. A new artificial joint can be implanted once the infection has been totally cleared. Patients with artificial joints must guard against infection for at least two years after their surgery by taking oral antibiotics before dental and urinary tract procedures. Even minor infections should be treated aggressively with antibiotics.

Conclusion

I started this book with the mention of some common myths people have about arthritis. I'd like to add two more.

The first is...

> "I can cure arthritis with natural methods only..."

The reality is:

- There is no cure for arthritis right now
- While natural methods are helpful... in fact, many medicines are derived from ingredients found in nature, they don't replace conventional therapies
- The best approach is a combination of alternative therapies and conventional therapies

The second myth, I'd like to bust is this...

> "Any doctor can treat arthritis..."

Since 1950, the amount of information a doctor has to know has increased more than 20 times!

You, as a patient, do not want to be a statistic!

Here's a fact... 98,000 Americans die every year from medical mistakes!

In fact, medical mistakes are the 8th leading cause of death in the United States... more than auto accidents, more than breast cancer, and more than AIDS!

www.arthritistreatmentcenter.com

These mistakes have two common causes:

- Lack of experience
- Lack of expertise

You are <u>29</u> times more likely to receive the right treatment with a board-certified rheumatologist.

And finally, the last myth…

"All rheumatologists are the same"

That's like saying all auto mechanics are the same… all electricians are the same… all financial consultants are the same, all attorneys are the same… all stock brokers are the same… You get the idea…

Insist on these prerequisites...

- American medical school graduate
- Board certification in rheumatology
- Passed rheumatology boards the first time – 21% don't!
- In practice a minimum of 15 years
- More than 60 publications in the scientific literature
- Active in clinical research

And these are the six qualities you should demand!

- Open-mindedness
- Empathy
- Experience in clinical practice
- Excellent reputation
- Top-notch facility and equipment
- Research experience

www.arthritistreatmentcenter.com

As I mentioned at the beginning, this book is not meant to be a comprehensive discussion of the topic of arthritis. For that, I refer you to my website http://www.arthritis-treatment-and-relief.com where you can obtain a copy of the excellent… and comprehensive Arthritis Treatment Kit.

I sincerely hope you've gotten a lot out of this book and I'd love to hear from you.

 You can reach me at nwei@arthritistreatmentcenter.com.

If you want to know more about Arthritis go to http://thebookonarthritis.com/arthritisbookoffer/ password: arthritis" for the Second Opinion Arthritis Treatment Kit (SOATK).

The definitive collection of information on both conventional and alternative therapies for arthritis. Here's some of what you'll discover…

- Discover 5 myths about arthritis that could cause you unnecessary vicious pain…
- Is it arthritis… is it bursitis… or tendonitis… the diagnosis is critical and here's why…
- Finger joint lumps and bumps… what are they?
- Foods to shun so you shrug off arthritis pain.
- The new super treatments that reverse rheumatoid arthritis.
- Best osteoarthritis remedy of all? This ultra-healing natural method stimulates self-repair!
- Common pain reliever, promoted as harmless, can trash your liver. Take it with alcohol… and die!
- Hocus-pocus magnet therapy? Discover the truth inside these pages.

Each chapter deals with a separate type of arthritis condition… and provides you with the information that will give you back your life.

Get 20% off the regular price of the SOATK.

Copy the following link on to your internet browser to take advantage of these incredible savings today!

http://thebookonarthritis.com/arthritisbookoffer/

password: arthritis

www.arthritistreatmentcenter.com

Made in the USA
Middletown, DE
13 March 2016